Walks around
... and over the

G000125396

Cover photograph: Fuller's Vale Pond, 2005

Walks around Headley
... and over the borders

ഗ ഗ ഗ

John Owen Smith

Walks around Headley ... and over the borders
First published July 2005, updated May 2010

Typeset and published by John Owen Smith
19 Kay Crescent, Headley Down, Hampshire GU35 8AH

Tel: 01428 712892
wordsmith@johnowensmith.co.uk
www.johnowensmith.co.uk

ISBN 978-1-873855-49-2

Printed and bound in Great Britain by CPI Antony Rowe, Chippenham and Eastbourne

Introduction

For several years there has been a booklet available describing the Footpaths, Bridleways and Byways of Headley parish. However it suffered from the very real problem that its world ended at the parish boundary, leaving walkers in limbo. They had either to retrace their steps, or boldly go into the unknown if they wished to complete a circular route.

This publication attempts to overcome that particular deficiency. It describes twelve circular walks which all start and end in Headley but which extend outside the hallowed borders of the parish – indeed outside the county and into Surrey and Sussex in some cases.

While the walks described here do not include every right of way in Headley parish, they do use most of them – and walkers may draw on the parish council booklet mentioned above to fill in the gaps if they wish.

We have also added historical information where appropriate, and photographs of features on the routes – some recent and some of past times.

We decided to use two start/finish points within the parish – the High Street for six routes at the western end (Walks 1–6), and the National Trust's small car park at the top of Pond Road for six routes towards the east (Walks 7–12).

On the western front we were delighted to be able to use the route of the Royal Woolmer Way, designed by Mike Wearing of the Deadwater Valley Trust, as a convenient outer boundary for our walks.

When compiling the overall map of our twelve walks it became clear, not only that the outline formed a rather pleasing shape (likened by some to a rose and by others to the face of a Pekinese dog!) but also that there was the possibility of forming an 'outer ring' route by linking the edges – hence the addition of linear Walk 13 (the 'missing link') to complete a ring of just over 20 miles.

For good measure we also include as Walk 14 the Flora Thompson Trail, a figure-of-eight walk between Grayshott and Griggs Green previously published in my book *On the Trail of Flora Thompson*, since it is largely within the area of the 'outer ring' and also provides a useful connection to the pubs of Liphook!

I cannot end without thanking my team of friends who tramped each path with me to check that the instructions made some sort of sense. I think we were all surprised to find such a diversity of scenery on our own doorstep.

So, I hope you enjoy the walks as much as we did. If you have any comments, adverse or admiring, please let me know.

John Owen Smith
May 2005

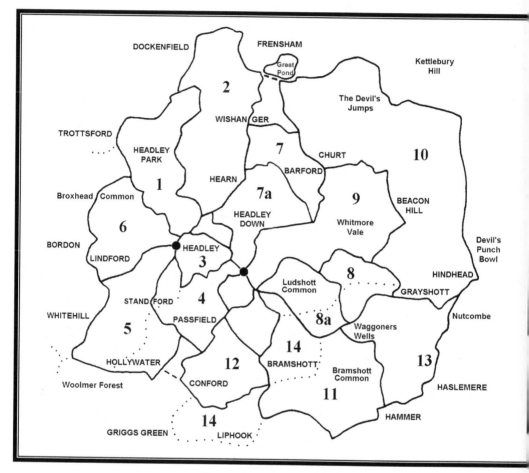

General map of the Walks

All of the walks will have muddy patches, some will have very muddy patches – waterproof footwear is recommended in all seasons.

Consult these texts for further information: *Footpaths, Bridleways and Byways of Headley Parish* for walks within Headley Parish boundaries, *To the Ar and Back* for a historic trail through Headley village and Arford, and *The Royal Woolmer Way* for the route around the western side of the outer ring.
See end of book for publishers.

The Walks

Ordnance Survey Explorer map 133 covers all but the northern-most parts of Walks 2 and 10 (it cuts off at Frensham Great Pond – the balance is covered by Explorer 145).

Note that where we use permissive paths rather than public rights of way, these may not always be clearly marked on the Ordnance Survey maps.

Map references: Headley High Street SU822362; Pond Road car park SU837356

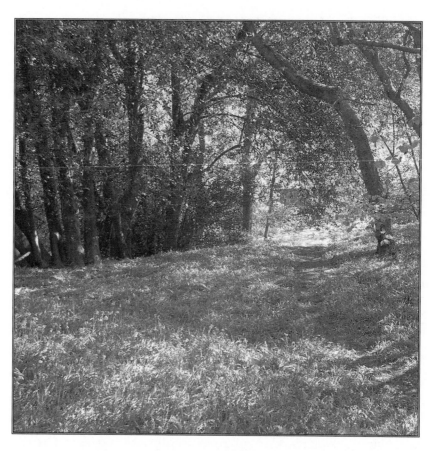

Bluebells near Huntingford Bridge – Walk 1

Walk 1 – Four Bridges

Distance approximately 6¼ miles/10km

The walk starts and ends in Headley High Street, visiting Trottsford, Cradle Lane, Dockenfield, Huntingford Bridge, Saunders Green, and The Hanger. It crosses the River Wey and the River Slea.

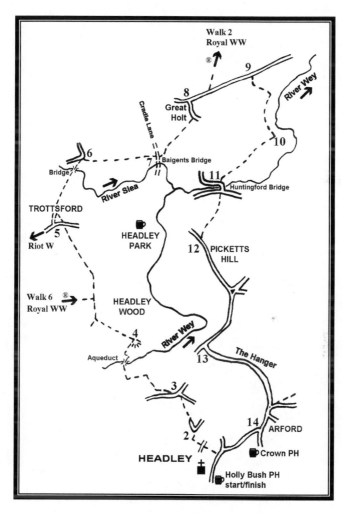

1　From the *Holly Bush*, turn right along Headley High Street, past the church and the old rectory, and just before *Belmont* take a path to the left. This crosses a road and then passes along two sides of the Holme School grounds, emerging on a road (Church Lane) at a right-angle bend.

> The Holme School takes its name from Dr George Holme, Rector of Headley 1718–65, who gave the parish a school in 1755. The original building stands beside the Village Green.

Church Lane takes its name from the fact that it forms part of the old track from Headley church towards the outlying parts of the parish on the way to Farnham. You will follow it, with some modern diversions, as far as Trottsford bridge.

2 Turn left along Church Lane (a cul-de-sac) and at its end pass through a footpath gate and downhill across fields. You emerge by *Huntingford Farm*, at the junction of Curtis Lane and Frensham Lane.

Huntingford Farm was built around 1774, according to a rent-roll of that date which has an entry for John Huntingford of: *"one close called Church-field with a tenement thereon newly erected containing 4 acres lying at Lackmore-cross on the south part of Curtis Lane"* – we assume it is this building. It was thatched until 1959, when the roof was lost in a fire. (You will encounter another Huntingford later in the walk – a confusing example of duplicate names in the parish).

3 The original route to Trottsford would have gone right and then left here, past Linsted Farm and Headley Wood Farm, but this is now closed as a right of way. Instead, turn left, following Frensham Lane towards Lindford for a short distance, then take the bridleway to the right, which follows the road uphill for a while before turning right, becoming rather rutted and narrow as it heads downhill between a hedge and a fence towards the river. After a left-hand bend, the track becomes considerably wider, then muddy as it passes through woodland which was once a watermeadow, to cross the River Wey by way of an old aqueduct (see below). It then zigzags sharply uphill.

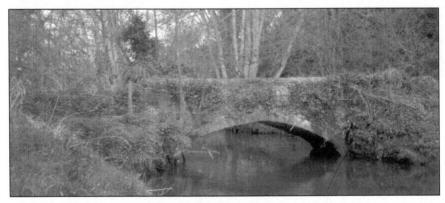

Aqueduct over the River Wey at Headley Wood

The aqueduct over the River Wey is part of an extensive system of channels which once extended along the river, through this parish and beyond, to regulate the watermeadows. Water was diverted from the river by a weir into a header ditch, which had a number of sluices along its length allowing water to be spread evenly over the meadow in a controlled fashion before draining back into the river. This system added nutrients to the land, allowing early crops of fodder to be produced, and a second cut to be made later in the year.

4 At the second gate, at the top of a rise, look back the way you have come – if the trees are not obscuring it, and if you know where to look, you may just make out the top of Headley Church tower nestling among the treetops. Here you rejoin the course of the original route before it was diverted. Turn left along the bridleway and after about half a mile follow it through a gate *(where **Walk 6** and the **Royal Woolmer Way** join us from the left)*, along a woodland track, past a Forestry Commission nursery, and uphill towards a road.

> On the ridge to your left just before reaching the road is a Bronze Age tumulus. There are several of these around the Woolmer Forest area.

*Note: The walk follows the **Royal Woolmer Way** to point 8.*

5 Cross the road and take the footpath ahead dipping across a field (the site of an old sandpit) then rising sharply to a stile. Turn right along a track, concreted at first through *Trottsford Farm*, which eventually crosses a stone bridge over the River Slea.

> The track through Trottsford Farm marks an old route to Farnham, prior to the building of the turnpike (now A325) around 1832, as indicated by the substantial nature of the bridge over the Slea. This bridge has no specific name in historical records as far as we can tell.

6 At a junction of tracks, take the footpath marked to the right which is routed around the forecourt of the sand-quarrying works and follow it beside the works road between a hedge and the sand pits to arrive at Cradle Lane (7).

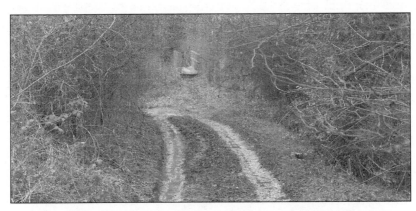

Cradle Lane with Baigents Bridge in the distance
– view from where Walks 1 & 2 cross Cradle Lane.

> According to legend, Cradle Lane is so named because the gypsies used a copse along it for their winter quarters, and the women gave birth to their babies in the Spring before setting out on their Summer travelling. There are tales of ghostly apparitions along this lane.

7 The third of the four bridges of the title is just down the lane to the right – it is known as Baigents Bridge and is now a footbridge next to a ford across the Slea – but our route does not lie in that direction. Instead, take the footpath

indicated on the other side of the lane and bear to the left (the path is not well defined) over a slight hill, across a ditch by a rubble 'bridge' and through a gap in a hedge directly ahead. It can be muddy here. Follow the field uphill (passing from Hampshire into Surrey) heading to the right of the half-timbered house (*Great Holt*), to a stile in the top corner of the field. Cross this, then another by a gate to a road. Turn left up the road to a triangular junction and turn right there (Old Lane).

> *Great Holt* was built on the site of an earlier farmhouse by Boyce Combe. During World War II the building was taken over as a girls' Convent which remained there until the 1980s.

8 *After about two hundred yards, **Walk 2** diverges on a footpath to the left.* Our walk continues along Old Lane for about half a mile, then takes a footpath to the right opposite Manor Farm (9).

> Look diagonally to your right as you walk down the road and you may see light aircraft using the Wishanger airstrip.

9 The path follows a farm track to a gate then cuts across an open field towards a distant hedge. Turn right at the hedge to follow a farm track in a left-handed curve through some gates (and back into Hampshire) with views across the Wey valley to your left. Just before the track emerges into an open field the right of way turns right up a track well-used by animals which soon becomes a path through light woodland.

10 This is a magnificent part of the walk in the bluebell season. After about half a mile the right of way turns left and descends by steps (take care) to a kissing gate, then across a field to meet a surfaced road near Huntingford Bridge (11).

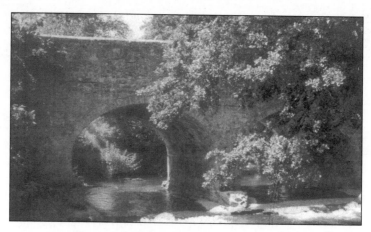

Huntingford Bridge over the River Wey

Huntingford Cottage and Forge, close to the bridge on the opposite side, go back into antiquity. The Collins family were blacksmiths here for many years, and at the autumn manoeuvres of 1874 we are told Dan Collins shoed a horse here for Prince Arthur, Duke of Connaught.

Today the forge is still used, though not for shoeing horses.

11 Turn left and go over the bridge to a T-junction. You now have the choice of footpath or bridleway to take you straight ahead up the opposite hill – either will bring you out on another surfaced road near Pickett's Hill Farm.

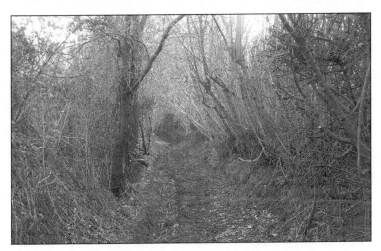

Bridleway up to Pickett's Hill.

12 Turn left and follow this road for about half a mile to a large green triangle (Saunders Green). Keep to the right-hand road, which descends past *Bayfields Farm* approaching the River Wey again (largely invisible through woodlands on the right), and turn left along The Hanger.

> The area round this junction was once known as Bilford (or Billyford), but the name now seems to have passed from living memory. On your left is *Hartfield House* where Commander Stephen King Hall lived during World War II – he was an MP, well-known radio commentator, and high on Hitler's most-wanted list.

13 Go along The Hanger and into the hamlet of Arford.

> There was once a sheep dip near to where the pumping station is now. Nearby was *The Wheatsheaf Inn*, demolished in 2001 (see photo p.18). The stream known locally as the Ar flows under the road here. Just upstream, at the bottom of Beech Hill Road, there is reputed to have been a tannery, which would have made the air in this part of the village less than salubrious at that time.

> Arford once contained several shops, but only *The Crown* public house remains now as a business (see photo p.26).

14 Turn right up Long Cross Hill to return to the High Street.
Note: The booklet 'To the Ar and Back' (published by The Headley Society) gives more details of the history of this area.

Walk 2 – To Frensham Great Pond and back

Distance approximately 8¾ miles/14km

This is an extension of Walk 1, taking in Dockenfield church, Frensham Mill, Frensham Great Pond, Wishanger and Hearn.

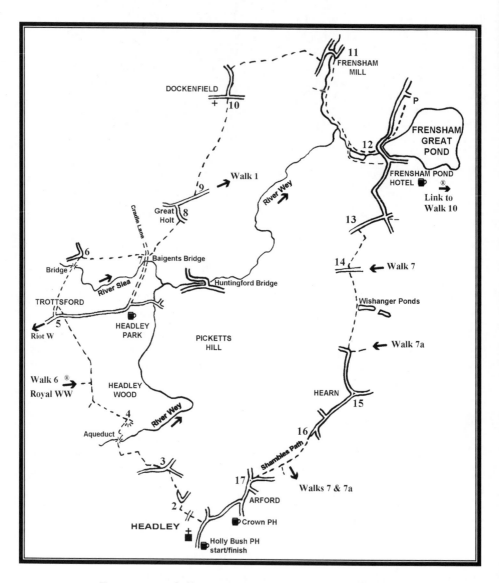

*For notes and illustrations up to point 8, see **Walk 1**.*

1 From the *Holly Bush*, turn right along Headley High Street, past the church and the old rectory, and just before *Belmont* take a path to the left. This

crosses a road and then passes along two sides of the Holme School grounds, emerging on a road (Church Lane) at a right-angle bend.

2 Turn left along Church Lane (a cul-de-sac) and at its end pass through a footpath gate and downhill across fields. You emerge by *Huntingford Farm*, at the junction of Curtis Lane and Frensham Lane.

3 Turn left, following Frensham Lane towards Lindford for a short distance, then take the bridleway to the right, which follows the road uphill for a while before turning right, becoming rather rutted and narrow as it heads downhill between a hedge and a fence towards the river. After a left-hand bend, the track becomes considerably wider, then muddy as it passes through woodland which was once a watermeadow, to cross the River Wey by way of an old aqueduct (see *Walk 1*). It then zigzags sharply uphill.

4 At its junction with a track at the top of a rise, turn left along the bridleway and after about half a mile follow it through a gate *(where **Walk 6** and the **Royal Woolmer Way** join us from the left)*, along a woodland track, past a Forestry Commission nursery, and uphill towards a road.

> As an alternative route from point 5 to point 7, turn right along the road passing Headley Park Hotel, follow the road as it bears left then take the track straight ahead (Cradle Lane) as the road bears right. Follow the track across the River Slea by footbridge (Baigents Bridge) to point 7.

5 *Note: The walk follows the **Royal Woolmer Way** to point 12.*
Cross the road and take the footpath ahead dipping across a field (the site of an old sandpit) to a stile. Turn right to join a track, concreted at first through *Trottsford Farm*, which eventually crosses a stone bridge over the River Slea.

6 At a junction of tracks, take the footpath marked to the right which is routed around the forecourt of the sand-quarrying works and follow it beside the works road between a hedge and the sand pits to arrive at Cradle Lane.

7 Take the footpath indicated on the other side of the lane and bear to the left (the path is not well defined) over a slight hill, across a ditch by a rubble 'bridge' and through a gap in a hedge directly ahead. It can be muddy here. Follow the field uphill heading to the right of the half-timbered house (*Great Holt*), to a stile in the top corner of the field. Cross this, then another by a gate to a road.

8 Turn left up the road to a triangular junction and turn right here (Old Lane).

9 After about a hundred yards along Old Lane, take a footpath to the left and follow it across a number of stiles and through a wood to Dockenfield (10).

> On a hill to the left of the path, Noel Coward owned a house briefly in 1924 where he wrote *Hay Fever* (allegedly in 3 days) and *Easy Virtue*.

> Dockenfield, though a tithing of the parish of Frensham, was considered part of Hampshire until 1895. The Church of the Good Shepherd here was built in 1910.

10 Cross the road, follow Bealswood Lane over a stream and turn right along a bridleway. Follow this to a road, turn left and then right down Mill Lane crossing the River Wey at Frensham Mill.

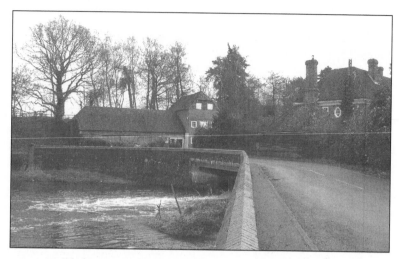

Bridge over the Wey at the site of Frensham Mill

Frensham Mill, or Beale's Mill, was one of several water mills on the southern River Wey. It stopped working in 1926.

11 At the Mill, turn right along a bridleway between the buildings. This follows the course of the river, passing a footbridge, and eventually bears left up a tributary stream. The right of way splits, a footpath to the right going round the other side of a small lake while the main track continues directly to meet a road at the edge of Frensham Great Pond (12).

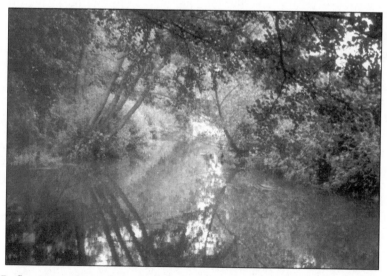

Reflections where the tributary from the Great Pond meets the river

Frensham Great Pond was constructed for the Bishop of Winchester as one of several fish ponds in his diocese, probably around AD 1200, by damming a stream forming the border between Surrey and Hampshire whose curved course still marked the county boundary through the pond until the boundary changes of 1991 put the whole pond in Surrey. *Frensham Pond Hotel* was known as the *White Horse Inn* until the beginning of the 20th century.

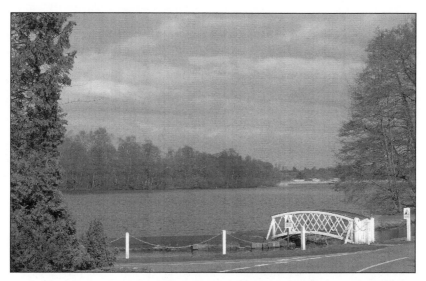

Frensham Great Pond from the Hotel

12 *Notes: The* **Royal Woolmer Walk** *turns left here to end at the Frensham Great Pond car park.*
   Link to **Walk 10** *and the '***outer ring***' by going along the south bank of the pond following the road passing the front of Frensham Pond Hotel.*
   Our walk turns right, along Bacon Lane. *This is narrow and traffic can travel at speed – please take care.* Follow the right-hand turn into Frensham Lane. After a quarter of a mile take the bridleway track on the left.

13 Follow the bridleway as it bears right and passes some new houses to meet another road. Cross straight over and follow the bridleway track opposite.

14 *Note:* **Walk 7** *joins here.*
   The track descends past *The Well House* and passes one of a chain of man-made ponds similar in size to Waggoners Wells but less well known (see photo p.40). It joins a road (Smithfield Lane) at a bend and we follow this for about half a mile to its junction with Churt Road at a grass triangle.

15 Turn right along Churt Road. *Keep eyes and ears open for approaching traffic.* Go past the entrance to Spats Lane on the right, then when the road bears left take the residential road straight ahead. This is Hearn Vale.

   Spats Lane is named after the spats worn by Walter Langrish who lived at the lower end of the lane at the end of the 19th century.

13 The road along Hearn Vale becomes a footpath which joins a road (Langton Drive) serving a number of properties in an area known as 'The Mount', before becoming a path again (known locally as 'Shambles Path').

Shambles is an old term for an area where animals were slaughtered. Since there is evidence of a tannery in Arford, we assume the deed was done here and the hides taken down the path for processing.

During the Second World War the field to the right of the path was the site of one of several army camps in the village and, from their War Diary, is thought to be the place where the Canadian Calgary Regiment was issued with the Churchill tanks which were later used on their ill-fated Dieppe raid.

17 At the junction of Barley Mow Hill and The Hanger we rejoin *Walk 1*, and return through Arford to Headley High Street.

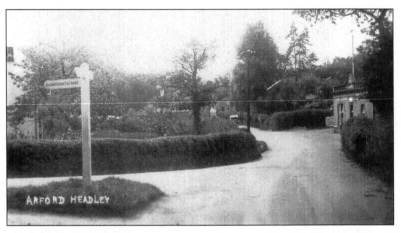

View from The Hanger/Barley Mow Hill junction along Arford Road in the early 20th century – note the Wheatsheaf Inn on the right, a site now redeveloped.

Walk 3 – Around Fuller's Vale

Distance approximately 2¾ miles/4.5km

This short walk starts and ends in Headley High Street, taking a tour past the old workhouse, through coppice woods behind Hilland, past the restored Fuller's Vale wildlife pond, over Headley Hill and along 'The Brae' footpath.

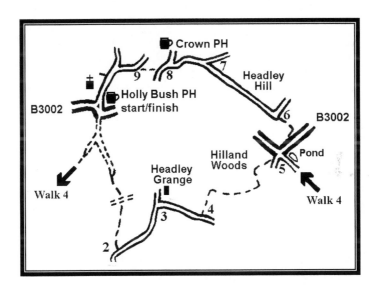

1 From the *Holly Bush*, turn left, cross the road and to the right of *Crabtree House* go along the lane called Headley Fields.

> Note the concrete surface at the beginning of Headley Fields – this was laid for the Canadian armoured regiments which used it during the Second World War as an entrance to a tank servicing facility.

Keep straight ahead at junctions – the lane becomes a footpath between hedges which eventually meets Liphook Road near an electricity sub-station.

> The bend on Liphook Road near where the path emerges was known in the past as 'Dirty Hole' corner, due to the pond which was there.

2 Turn left along the road (taking care of traffic) and in about a quarter of a mile take Hurland Lane to the right (3).

> Near the junction with Hurland Lane is *Headley Grange* which from 1795 to 1871 was the Workhouse of the parishes of Bramshott, Headley and Kingsley. In November 1830 a mob of several hundred sacked the house, an incident for which seven men were transported to Australia. In the 1970s it was used as a recording studio, most famously by Led Zeppelin who recorded their hit 'Stairway to Heaven' there.

3 Follow Hurland Lane up the hill for about two hundred yards to the end of

19

the field on the left (4).

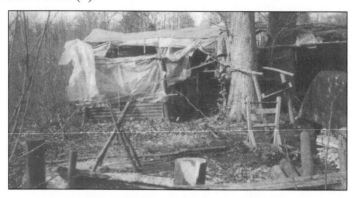

Coppice-worker's camp in Hilland Woods, 1991

Hilland Woods contains chestnut coppice, a crop which has been cut traditionally on a ten-year cycle to obtain wooden poles. These have many uses in agriculture and the garden, for fences, furniture, etc.

4 Take the Public Bridleway which follows the edge of the wood, with the field on the left and coppice wood on the right. At a T-junction, turn right at a guide post and follow the bridleway as it takes a generally 'D-shaped' course through the woods following an earth bank on the left and flanked by rhododendrons in places. About a hundred yards after a usually particularly muddy patch, look for another guide post pointing right and take this track which eventually drops sharply downhill through holly trees to Fullers Vale pond.

The pond was restored in 2003 having been drained thirty years previously during flood-prevention works. It is fed by underground springs and has now been designated a 'wildlife' pond, its plant and animal life being left to develop naturally (see photo on front cover).

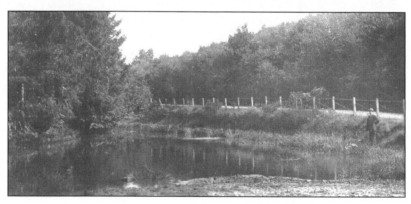

Fullers Vale pond before the First World War

5 Cross the main road with care at the four-way junction and walk along the left-hand side of Beech Hill to take the bridleway which passes *Oakdene* and climbs straight ahead uphill. Follow the track as it bends to the left and

meets concrete at Headley Hill Road.

> As with the concrete found at the start of the walk, this too was laid by the Canadian forces during World War II to prevent track-laying vehicles from tearing up the road surface. Tanks and troops were billeted under trees along the right-hand side of the road during the years before D-Day.

6 Continue straight ahead along the road, which becomes more pitted as it descends to meet a surfaced road (Bowcot Hill).

> On the left, hidden by shrubs, the land falls away into Fullers Vale. In the past this bank was worked for fuller's earth, used in fulling mills which we know existed locally on the River Wey. Of the houses along here, the history of *Windridge* has been documented in a local book, and *Benifold*, built in 1899, has been both a religious retreat and the home of the pop group Fleetwood Mac – it is now a private house.

7 Turn left down Bowcot Hill which crosses the Ar stream then rises to meet Arford Road by the gate to *Arford House*.

> Downstream of the bridge over the Ar there used to be a pond in which troops on manoeuvres from Bordon to Ludshott Common watered their horses.

8 Turn left up Arford Road keeping your ears open for traffic approaching round the blind corner, and shortly take the steps up to the right. Follow the footpath across a drive and between properties built in an old gravel quarry on the left and the old Manse on the right to join a road (Long Cross Hill) opposite *Medway* which was once the post office and bank.

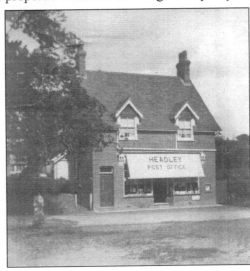

> The footpath is known as the 'Brae', so-named by American author Brett Harte when he stayed as a visitor at Arford House in the late 19th century.
>
> Just above the steps there used to be a bridge, built in 1921, carrying the drive to *Kirklands* over the path, but it disappeared some years ago.

9 Turn left up Long Cross Hill and left again at the top to return to the High Street.

Old post office & bank in Long Cross Hill

Walk 4 – Down by the Riverside

Distance approximately 5 miles/8km

This walk starts and ends in Headley High Street, visiting Standford, following the River Wey upstream through Passfield to *Waterside*, then via High Hurlands and Ludshott Common to Fullers Vale where it rejoins Walk 3 in returning over Headley Hill to the High Street.

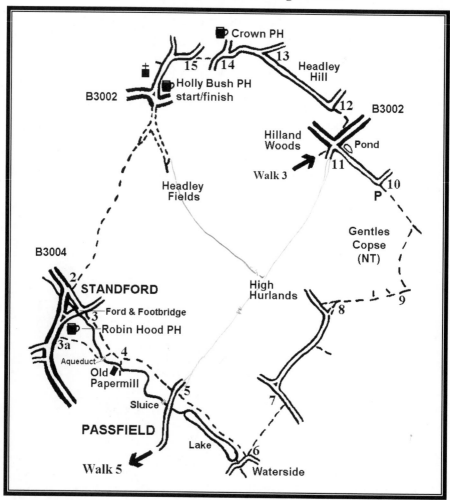

1 From the *Holly Bush*, turn left, cross the road with care and to the right of *Crabtree House* go along the lane called Headley Fields. After a hundred yards or so, fork right by *Mayfield House* along another unpaved lane. Keep to the footpath where this divides to the left. After passing between hedges, it crosses fields through a number of 'kissing gates' and eventually descends to meet a road (Tulls Lane) at Standford.

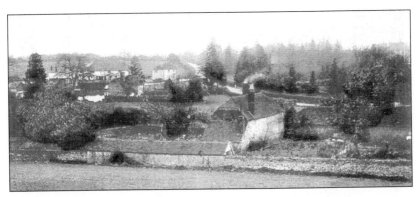

View over Standford in 1903 taken from near the footpath from Headley

2 Turn left along Tulls Lane. Where it bends sharply left, take the footpath passing through a gate and garden straight ahead. (To the right at this point is a footbridge over the River Wey leading to Standford Village Green and the *Robin Hood* pub, see photo p.28).

> The ford and bridge here have been favourite subjects for artists and photographers through the years. The ford is not recommended for car users! Downstream of the bridge the wooded area was once the mill pond for Standford Paper Mill, which shut down around 1886.

For an interesting diversion, go over the bridge and past the Robin Hood – take a path to the left (at 3a on map opposite) at a sign showing Open Access information and go through a kissing gate into old watermeadows. Make your way through the meadow to an aqueduct (rebuilt in 2006) where you can cross the river again and rejoin the walk between Points 3 and 4.

3 Follow the track through the garden, then between fences. The field to the right which falls towards the river is a nature reserve (old watermeadow).

4 Ignoring a flat concrete bridge over the river to the right, carry straight on following the footpath along the river bank.

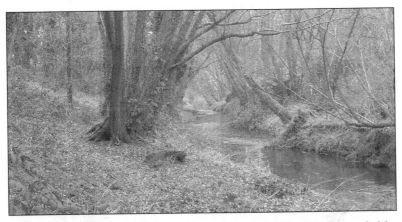

Footpath beside the River Wey between Standford and Passfield

The buildings opposite used to be Bramshott Paper Mill, closed in 1924. Now the site and the area of the old mill pond is used by a variety of light industrial and commercial operations.

This path is a pretty, shaded walk along the bank of the River Wey. It emerges up a sharp incline to meet an unmade lane serving houses which leads shortly to a surfaced road.

Walk 5 leaves us here.

Nearby to the right is a good example of a sluice which diverted water from the river as part of the water meadow irrigation system which once ran along both sides of the river. It can be seen from the road bridge (see photo p.28).

5 Cross the road diagonally, passing to the right of a gate and following the path along the bank of a lake formed from damming the river. At the other end of the lake you arrive at a crossing of public rights of way at *Waterside*.

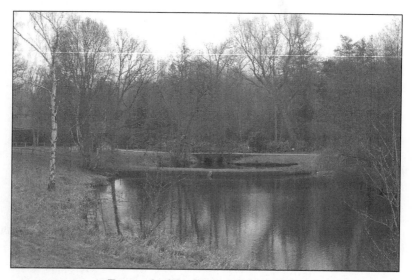

Top end of the lake at 'Waterside'

In the private grounds at 'Waterside', water from the river is pumped into side channels or 'leats' which run at a higher level. These, once part of the water meadow irrigation system, now act as a supply for water features in the garden.

6 Take the bridleway on the left to meet a road (Bramshott Lane).
7 Turn left along the road, then shortly right along Gentles Lane which soon becomes a 'sunken lane' climbing uphill.

Sunken lanes are a feature of this part of Hampshire. In places here the activity of burrowing animals often shifts quantities of the bank soil down onto the road surface.

8 Where the lane bends left, take the muddy bridleway straight ahead, turning right shortly where it joins another bridleway known locally as Roman Road.

Follow this (waterproof footwear recommended) until you see a National Trust sign for Gentles Copse on the left.

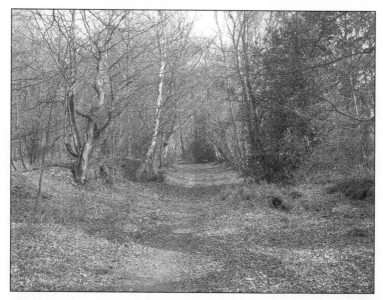

'Roman Road' – bridleway from High Hurlands to Ludshott Common

Local legend says that this track was used by Roman soldiers on their way to cross the river at Standford. It is known that in Roman times Gentles Copse was coppiced for the manufacture of charcoal.

9 There are several paths from here which cross the Trust land to arrive at the bridleway leading to Pond Road car park. To follow the marked public right of way, carry on along the bridleway for another quarter of a mile or so and take a bridleway sharp left and uphill. This follows a firebreak between woods over a rise and descends into a valley (follow the overhead electric cables). Join the main track along the valley bottom near an old concrete dam, turning left to reach the NT car park in just over a quarter of a mile.

During the Second World War, army training activities with tracked vehicles denuded Ludshott Common of most of its vegetation – as a result, when it rained water poured off the Common instead of being absorbed, ran down this valley as a river and flooded properties in Fullers Vale and in Arford. Some concrete flood prevention works can still be seen here and there in the undergrowth.

10 Carry on down the valley (along Pond Road) to Fullers Vale pond.
*This is point 5 of **Walk 3**, which you follow in returning to your start point. See notes and illustrations at p.20.*

11 Cross the main road with care at the four-way junction and walk along the left-hand side of Beech Hill to take the bridleway which passes *Oakdene* and climbs straight ahead uphill. Follow the track as it bends to the left and meets concrete at Headley Hill Road.

12 Continue straight ahead along the road, which becomes more pitted as it descends to meet a surfaced road (Bowcot Hill).

13 Turn left down Bowcot Hill to cross the Ar stream and then rise to meet Arford Road by the gate to Arford House. (Note that *The Crown* public house with its secluded garden is conveniently just down the road to your right).

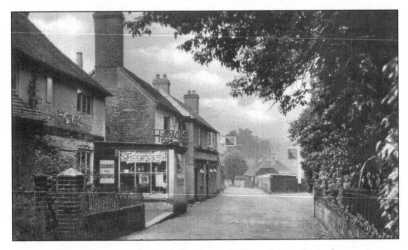

The Crown Inn at Arford, with shop in earlier days

Note: The booklet 'To the Ar and Back' (published by The Headley Society) gives more details of the history of this area.

14 Turn left up Arford Road keeping your ears open for traffic approaching round the blind corner, and shortly take the steps up to the right. Follow the footpath across a drive and between properties built in an old gravel quarry on the left and the old manse on the right to arrive at a road (Long Cross Hill) opposite *Medway*.

15 Turn left up Long Cross Hill and left again at the top to return to the High Street.

Walk 5 – To the Military railway

Distance approximately 7¾ miles/12.5km

This walk starts and ends in Headley High Street, visiting Standford, Passfield Common, Woolmer Forest, the track of the Longmoor Military Railway, Walldown earthworks, Deadwater Valley and Headley Mill.

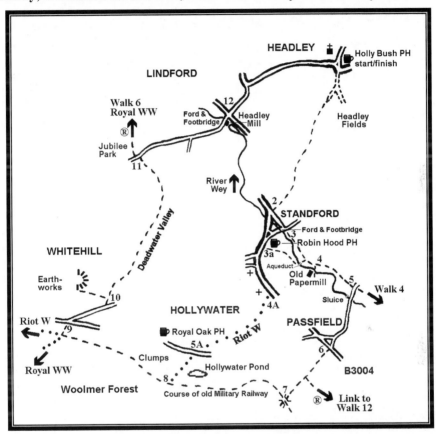

*For notes and illustrations up to point 5, see **Walk 4**.*

1   From the *Holly Bush*, turn left, cross the road with care and to the right of Crabtree House go along the lane called Headley Fields. After a hundred yards or so, fork right by *Mayfield House* along another unpaved lane. Keep to the footpath where this divides to the left. After passing between hedges, it crosses fields through a number of 'kissing gates' and eventually descends to meet a road (Tulls Lane) at Standford.

2   Turn left along Tulls Lane. Where it bends sharply left, take the footpath passing through a gate and garden straight ahead. (To the right at this point is a footbridge over the River Wey leading to Standford Village Green and the Robin Hood pub, and to the **Rioters' Walk**).

27

*Part of the **Rioters' Walk** can be used as a short-cut here if desired, but be prepared for boggy terrain – see p.32 for details.*

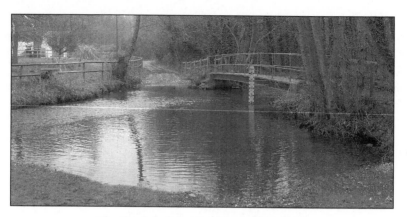

The ford and footbridge at Standford

3   Follow the track through the garden, then between fences. The field to the right which falls towards the river is a nature reserve (old watermeadow).

4   Ignoring a flat concrete bridge over the river to the right, carry straight on following the footpath along the river bank. This path is a pretty, shaded walk along the bank of the River Wey. It emerges up a sharp incline to meet an unmade lane serving houses which leads shortly to a surfaced road. (You may alternatively follow the river bank, turning right just before the end of the path to pass a sign indicating a nature reserve – this route passes the old sluice-bridge before emerging at the road).

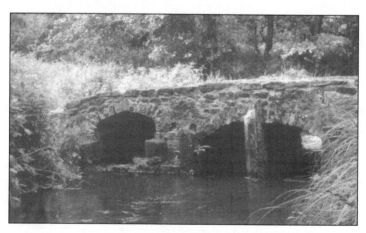

Passfield Sluice-bridge

The sluice diverted water from the river as part of the water meadow irrigation system which ran along both sides of the river.

5   Turn right along the road to cross the River Wey and arrive at Passfield Common.

The triangular green in front of the houses at Passfield belongs to the National Trust and is part of a larger area owned by them on the other side of the main road. It is often left untended as part of the Trust's planned management of wildlife areas.

6   Cross the B3004 and take the track to the left of the large white building (which was once the *Passfield Oak* hotel). Continue along the track which becomes a path and follow it down to cross a stream (where it can be muddy) before arriving at a dismantled railway bridge where the line of the old military railway crossed on an embankment.
*Note: The link from **Walk 12** joins from the left before you cross the stream.*
The railway was constructed in a loop around Woolmer Forest by the Army in order to instruct soldiers on how to operate (and if necessary destroy) railway systems. It closed in 1969.

Of greater antiquity is the site of a hunting lodge (Linchborough) used by monarchs from the time of Edward I – this now lies within the military danger area. Woolmer Forest is a haven for many rare forms of wildlife – one benefit of the military occupation of the land.

7   A permissive path follows the line of the old railway, which is outside the boundary of the military 'danger area'. Go under the bridge hole, turn right and follow the track up an incline to join the course of the old railway track.

To the right of the track the land falls towards Hollywater Pond (out of sight behind trees), restored in recent years by the National Trust and said to be the site of a leper colony in ancient times.

8   *After about three-quarters of a mile, the short-cut via the **Rioters' Walk** rejoins us along a grass track to the right of a house.*
Continue along the 'railway track'. Shortly, on the right, look for the fallen remains of an old wooden railway viaduct which the Army would build and destroy for practice. Soon after this the track divides – take the right fork uphill. This forestry road runs in a fairly straight 'switchback' line over the shoulders of a couple of wooded hills.

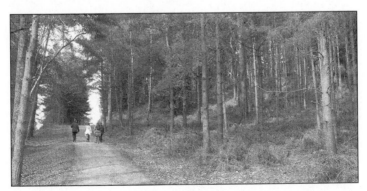

Climbing the forestry road beside Hollywater Clump

The wooded hill 'clumps' are associated in legend with burials from the leper colony, but most evidence points to them being of natural origin.

About three-quarters of a mile after the fork, look for a track to the right. This leads you to a road (Liphook Road). Depending on which of several tracks you have taken, you may emerge opposite the junction of this road with Walldown Road, or you may have to walk along the verge to find this junction.

9 *Note: The walk from here to point 11 follows the* **Royal Woolmer Way***.*

Follow Walldown Road for about a quarter of a mile until you see the Deadwater Valley Local Nature Reserve sign on the left. Turn into the wood here. This part of the walk is on a permissive path through land managed by the Deadwater Valley Trust.

You may like to make a short diversion to visit the Walldown earthworks – shortly after entering the wood take the track rising to the left beside a fence bordering school grounds on the right. After a stiff climb, enter the enclosure by way of a stile where there is a notice giving a brief history of the site. There are views to the east from the top. Retrace your steps downhill to continue the walk.

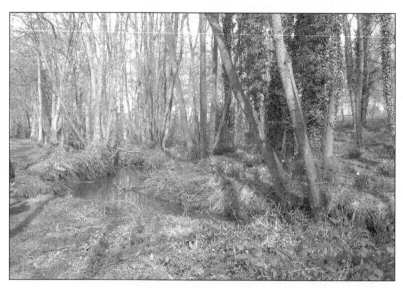

The Deadwater Valley

10 Follow the well-used path through the woods ignoring paths to residential roads on the left. Cross a driveway and continue along the woodland path which eventually passes Knox's Pond on the left before running close to the Deadwater Stream on the right. Keep the stream on your right until reaching a footbridge which crosses over. Cross the bridge and turn immediately left along the bank of the stream to meet Mill Chase Road.

11 Turn right along Mill Chase Road and, after passing one school on the left and two on the right, you arrive at Headley Mill. Here the road fords the River Wey at the mill's tailrace; you may cross by the footbridge.

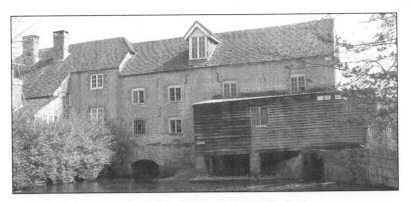

Rear of Headley Mill from the ford

Headley Mill has been said to be the last commercially working water mill in Hampshire. There has been a mill here since the time of Domesday. The workings inside are not generally open to the public.

11 Cross the B3004 and go along Mill Lane, directly opposite the ford. At its junction with Headley Road turn right to climb the hill and return to Headley.

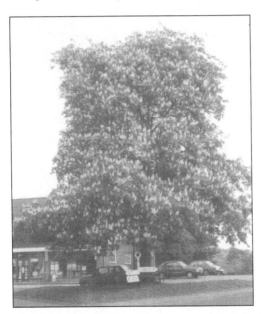

The Chestnut Tree at Headley, taken in May 1991

Short-cut via the Rioters' Walk

*Follow **Walk 5** to point 3.*

A3 Cross the River Wey using the footbridge, and follow the road from the ford as it passes in front of the *Robin Hood* pub (changed in 2010 to a restaurant) to join the main road (B3004). Follow the verge path up the hill and pass both the Gospel Hall and the Methodist Church on the right.

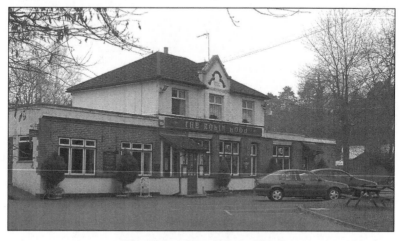

The Robin Hood, Standford

A4 Look for a path on the right leading to a kissing gate into National Trust land – part of Passfield Common fenced to keep grazing animals from straying. Head in a generally south-west direction across the common to find a kissing gate in the perimeter fence on the south side at the side of a road. *Be warned – there are no designated paths and it can be extremely boggy in places.* For those with GPS, start at SU81538 34169 and end at SU 80962 33667.

A5 Turn right along the road. After a while (the distance depends on which gate you used out of the Common) take the track on the left leading to a Builders' Merchant. *(You may continue up the road for a further 300 yards to visit the Royal Oak pub if you wish, and then either proceed further up the road to rejoin the **Walk 5** at point 9, or retrace your steps to carry on here).*

An interesting diversion down paths to the left of the track takes you to the edge of Hollywater Pond, restored by the National Trust.

Follow the track across a stream and past the Builders' Merchant, then take the path to the left of *Stone Cottage*. This leads up to the old railway track, rejoining **Walk 5** at point 8 (see p.29).

Walk 6 – Right round Lindford

Distance approximately 5 miles/8km

This walk starts and ends in Headley High Street, visiting Headley Mill, Bordon Inclosure, Broxhead Common and Headley Wood aqueduct.

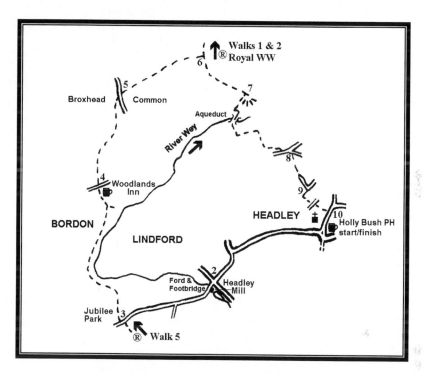

1 From the *Holly Bush*, take Mill Lane (B3002) directly ahead. Follow it downhill and turn left at its junction at the bottom of the hill. You soon meet the B3004 at a crossroads. Opposite is Headley Mill with its roving geese.

Headley Mill has been said to be the last commercially working water mill in Hampshire. There has been a mill here since the time of Domesday. The workings inside are not generally open to the public.

2 Take the road directly ahead, which fords the River Wey at the mill's tailrace (see photo p.31). You may cross by the footbridge. Follow the road away from the river and towards the centre of Bordon, passing schools to left and right. Soon after crossing the Deadwater stream, turn right into Jubilee Park.

The town of Bordon has developed from an Army Camp which was started in the early 20th century following the Boer Wars. Before that it was a sparsely-populated area, part of Woolmer Forest.

Note: The walk from here to point 6 follows the **Royal Woolmer Way**. *Some of the route is on permissive rather than public paths.*

3 Cross the park aiming for the end of the houses on the left. Go round the end

gardens keeping to the left (don't go down tracks to the river bank) noting the small square MoD boundary stone at the corner of the gardens.

The path crosses a buried water pipe then descends to cross a small stream. At a fork of tracks, keep right and pass under electric cables to meet another track coming from the right – then at a crossroads of tracks (with an exit to housing ahead in the distance) turn right along a track which is surfaced in parts. Follow this until it exits into a housing estate. Turn right to skirt round the end house and follow the path into the woods.

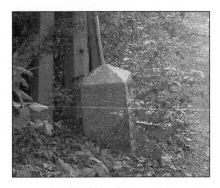

MoD Boundary stone

This area is called Bordon Inclosure and was once the site of a royal hunting lodge.

Look for a path to the right which crosses an 'orange' ditch. After this, a fairly indistinct path leading off at a diagonal to your left brings you eventually to a cobbled path. Turn left on this to arrive at *Woodlands Inn* on Lindford Road.

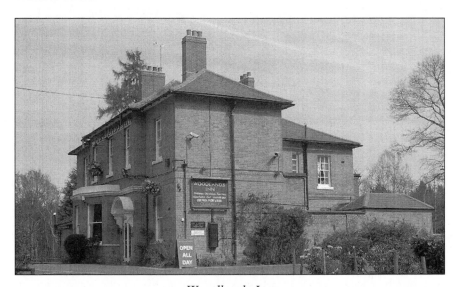

Woodlands Inn

Woodlands Inn was once an officers' mess, and then became the only pub in Bordon – it is said that in the past the Army forbade pubs to be opened within a certain radius of the Camp.

4   Cross Lindford Road and follow the public footpath straight ahead. The path rises, passing St Lucia House on the left. Keep ahead up the hill. Just before the top, bear right and follow the sandy track as it curves to the left. Head for

high ground when tracks diverge – you will arrive at a pool in an old sandpit. Turn right to skirt the edge of the pool, climbing a steep, loose sand path to arrive at Broxhead Farm Road (B3004).

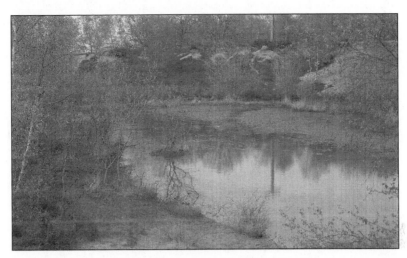

Sandpit Pond, Broxhead Common

5   Cross the road with care (fast traffic comes over the brow from the left) and take the public footpath opposite which crosses the unenclosed eastern part of Broxhead Common and then runs between fences and hedges (good for blackberrying in season) through fields. There are views to right and left. The path goes downhill to meet the old Church path from Headley.

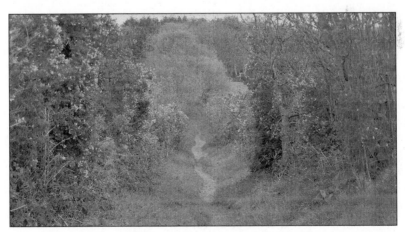

Path from Broxhead Common

There was a confrontation on Broxhead East Common one Saturday evening in 1973 when about two miles of landowner's fence was removed in order to reinforce a successful claim of commoners' rights.

6   Leaving the gate to the left at this junction, turn right along the track towards

Headley *(following the outward leg of **Walk 1** in reverse).*

7 After about half a mile the right of way turns right through a gate (avoiding the 'strictly private' Headley Wood Farm) and after another gate zigzags downhill to cross the River Wey over an old aqueduct. The track then passes through woodland where it can be muddy. Soon after leaving this it becomes rather rutted and narrow for a while as it heads uphill between a hedge and a fence. Eventually it falls to join Frensham Lane. Turn left past *Huntingford Farm* and its barn to the junction with Curtis Lane.

See notes on p.10 relating to the aqueduct and Huntingford Farm.

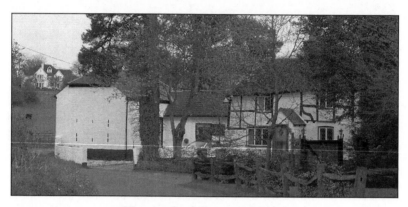

Huntingford Farm and Barn

8 Cross the stile by the gate to the left of *Huntingford Farm* barn, take the footpath leading diagonally uphill across fields, and enter Church Lane through a kissing gate.

9 At the bend in Church Lane take the footpath to the right. This skirts the playing field of the Holme School, crosses a road and passes the end of the churchyard before reaching the High Street by the entrance to *Belmont*.

Belmont once belonged to the Army, and still has a War Department boundary stone at its gate (one of four originally marking the four corners of the WD property).

10 Turn right along the High Street to return to the village centre.

Walk 7 – The Hampshire/Surrey border

Distance approximately 6½ miles/10.5km (option 5½ miles/8.8km)

This walk starts and ends at the National Trust car park in Pond Road, visiting Openlands, Hammer Lane, Whitmore Vale, Barford Mills, Churt, Symondstone, Wishanger, Hearn, Arford Common and Fullers Vale. *There is a shorter route offered between Hammer Lane and Hearn, visiting Assisi, Plaster Hill Farm and Park Lane – see Walk 7a.*

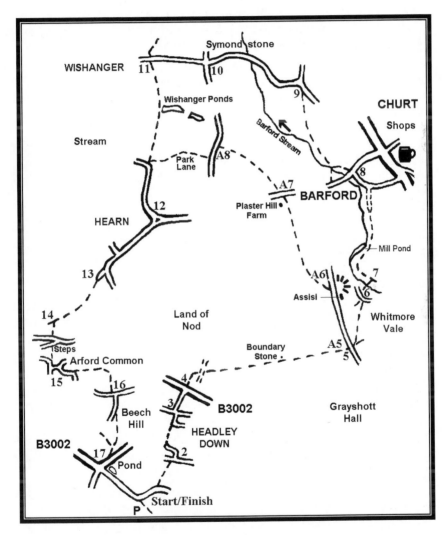

1 From the car park, follow Furze Hill Road uphill – where it bends to the right, keep straight ahead on a deep-rutted footpath climbing through woods known as 'Openlands'. Follow this in a more-or-less straight line to emerge at a junction of unmade roads.

Note the plaque in the ground to the right of the path as you approach the road. The 10 acres of 'Openlands' was bought by Dr Elizabeth Wilks (who died in 1953) and is managed for the benefit of local residents by the Headley Public Utility Society.

2   Cross straight over into Oakhill Road – follow this as it bends to the left, and at its dead end take the footpath to the right and downhill between fence and hedge to join Linden Road as it descends to the bottom of the valley.

3   Turn left along Honeysuckle Lane and very soon right, up the steep Wilsons Road to meet Grayshott Road (4).

Wilsons Road is named after the family who ran the first post office and telephone exchange in Headley Down from their shop, now a private house *The Village Store* at the junction with Fairview Road.

4   Look for a public footpath sign on the opposite side of the road – take this path, which follows inside the boundary of the housing estate, crossing the end of a cul-de-sac before exiting through a gap in the fence at the bottom left hand corner almost hidden by a garden wall. Bear right to cross a tarmac drive (to the *Land of Nod*) and go through a wooden barrier opposite to follow the footpath on the other side. This proceeds in a fairly straight line through woods, passing paddocks on the right and some clear land on the left before descending a steep-sided valley. Just before the bottom, it used to pass a flat cross-shaped stone, now sadly missing, laid in the ground on the left-hand side of the path to mark a corner of the boundary agreed in

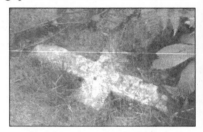

Stone marked the location and direction of the Grayshott/Headley boundary

1921 between Headley and Grayshott civil parishes. Cross a private track along the valley bottom, then ascend even more steeply up the other side, maintaining a straight line until you reach a road (Hammer Lane).

The direction of this long, straight path as shown on maps lines up almost exactly with Headley Church – is this significant? Another mystery is the name Hammer Lane – normally this relates to hammer ponds or ironworks but no such activities seem to have existed here.

5   *The shorter* **Walk 7a** *diverges here – see step A5 on p.42.*
Cross Hammer Lane and take the footpath diagonally to the left which descends through woods to Whitmore (or Whitmoor) Vale Road. Turn left for a short distance, then take the footpath to the right.

Whitmore Vale was once an area known for its 'squatters cottages': *"These were erected during the night, trees cut down to form the framework, the walls being made of turf and the roof thatched with heather. Before morning wives and children were installed as the law would not allow the bailiffs to remove the roof of a house containing children. On being thus occupied for a certain time the cabin and land on which it stood could be claimed."— Mrs W.E. Belcher, 1925.*

6   The path descends through a landscaped area to cross the stream on a bridge made of railway sleepers. This is the county boundary between Hampshire and Surrey. Go through a gate and climb the steep path on the other side to meet a track running along the Surrey side of the valley.

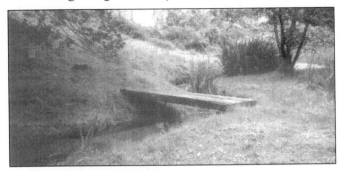

Crossing the county border in Whitmore Vale

7   Turn left along the track, which soon runs between iron fences and descends towards Barford passing mill ponds and the sites of three old water mills. Towards the bottom it joins a surfaced road (Kitts Lane) before arriving at Barford Bridge where Churt Road crosses the stream (8).

> Of the three mills here, the upper and lower ones made paper and the middle one (much the oldest, and generally known as Barford Mill) ground corn. The structure of the upper mill no longer exists (the 'Barracks Cottages' were built from its stones) but its mill pond known locally as Power's Pond remains a feature. The middle mill survives, sympathetically converted to a private house. The three-storey building at the site of the lower mill (now called *The Old Mill*) remains.

For those requiring sustenance, the shops and pub at Churt crossroads are a mere couple of hundred yards away, up the road to the right.

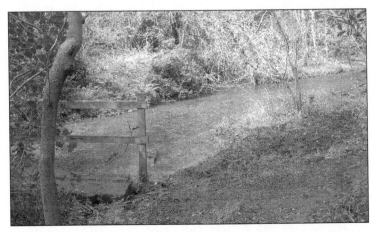

Footbridge and ford at bottom of Ivy House Lane

39

8 Cross Churt Road and take the footpath by the water pumping station. This first rises then descends to meet the stream again at a footbridge and ford. Do not cross the stream but turn right to follow the track, which climbs past *Ivy House Cottage* to meet Lampard Lane near *Barford Court.*

> At the beginning of the 20th century *Barford Court* was the home of George Murray, a Professor of Greek at Oxford and friend of George Bernard Shaw who lived in Hindhead at the time.

9 Turn left into Lampard Lane, then shortly left again to Symondstone (or Simmonstone) returning to Hampshire as you cross the stream. The road meets Bacon Lane at a crossroads.

> Simmonstone is named after the Seman family who owned property here in the 13th century – Seman's Stone, which was taken away some time after 1950, marked a point on the boundary of the Manor of Wishanger, at one time held by a Seman. Bacon Lane is named after the Bacon family – Roger Bacoun is mentioned in a Winchester Pipe Roll entry for Headley as early as 1320.

10 Cross over Bacon Lane and go straight ahead along Wishanger Lane until just beyond some buildings where a bridleway crosses.

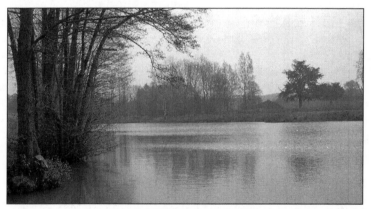

One of the Wishanger ponds

11 Turn left. The track descends past *The Well House* which is thought to be the site of the old manor house of Wishanger manor (note also the old vineyard on the right). The valley below contains a string of man-made ponds, and the track passes the end of one, used for fishing, before joining a road (Smithfield Lane) at a bend (*Walk 7a rejoins here*) – follow this for about half a mile to its junction with Churt Road at a grass triangle.

12 Turn right along Churt Road. *Keep eyes and ears open for approaching traffic.* Go past the entrance to Spats Lane on the right, then when the road bears left take the residential road straight ahead. This is Hearn Vale.

13 The road along Hearn Vale becomes a footpath which joins a road (Langton Drive) serving a number of properties before becoming a path again. *See notes on pp.17/18.*

14 At the end of a paddock, take a footpath to the left which descends to a road (Barley Mow Hill). Turn left, and shortly sharp right up the unmade track called Arford Common, then soon take a flight of steps on the left by the side of a house – these lead to a narrow path between a hedge and a fence which emerges at another track. Follow the track uphill.

15 At a junction at the top of the hill, take a rough track to the left, still climbing, past the end of the terrace of houses known as Fairview Terrace. At the top of the rise the track splits, going either side of a wooded area. Take the right-hand fork and soon, where this bears sharply right, carry straight on along a level path soon passing a grass area on the left. The path rises gently through the woods of Arford Common. At a junction near the top, bear right to pass a fixed metal

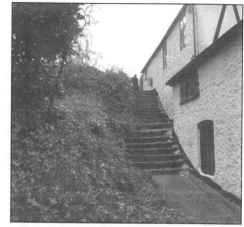

Steps at Arford Common

barrier giving access to a long, straight path between a hedge and fence meeting a road at a second barrier.

16 Turn left, then right (opposite the Scout Hut) into Headley Hill Road. There are still signs of concrete roads from wartime tank activity here. When woodland starts on the left, take the public footpath which cuts diagonally through the woods. Follow this, turning hard right by a concrete fence post at a corner of a garden then straight on where it crosses another footpath, to its junction with a bridleway which descends to meet a main road (Beech Hill) near the pond in Fullers Vale (see notes and picture p.20).

17 Cross the main road with care, and follow Pond Road alongside the pond to return to the National Trust car park.

ⓛⓛⓛ

Walk 7a – Assisi, Plaster Hill and Park Lane

A5 *Follow* **Walk 7** *to point 5.*

Turn left along Hammer Lane for a few hundred yards, passing houses on the right until arriving at the drive to *Assisi*. There is a good view across Whitmore Vale and beyond from here.

Assisi was once known as *Llanover* and in the early 20th century was the home of the Prichards who were benefactors in Churt. More recently it was a maternity home for unmarried mothers, run by Catholic nuns from the Cenacle Convent in Grayshott – it is now a private house.

A6 Take the footpath opposite *Assisi*, crossing a stile and keeping to the right at a fork. The path is soon flanked by holly, then descends gently becoming a typical 'sunken lane' with interesting plant and animal life. It emerges on the drive to *Coombe Farm* which in turn meets Churt Road near *Plaster Hill Farm*.

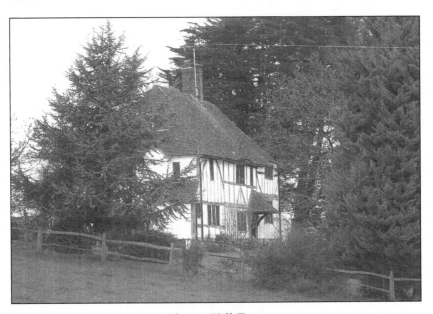

Plaster Hill Farm

Plaster Hill Farm was called *Luke's* on copyhold documents many years ago, possibly from the surname Lucas. The first marriage recorded in the Headley parish register on 1st July 1539 was between Robert Hardyng of 'Playstow hill' and Kateryn Woolffe.

A7 At Churt Road take the footpath opposite. This crosses several stiles and fields before passing through a wood in a valley (it can be wet underfoot as springs rise here) and arriving at a road (Bacon Lane).

Bacon Lane is named after the Bacon family, Roger Bacoun being mentioned in a Winchester Pipe Roll entry for Headley as early as 1320.

A8 Turn left along the road, and shortly take a wide and well-maintained bridleway to the right – this is known as Park Lane. In about a quarter of a mile, on the left just before a bend, fans of 'Monopoly' will be glad to see that there is a link constructed for horse riders to travel between Park Lane and Mayfair (riding stables). In another quarter of a mile we come to a junction of bridleways (*and rejoin* **Walk 7** *here*). Turn left onto a road (Smithfield Lane) and follow this for about half a mile to its junction with Churt Road at a grass triangle.

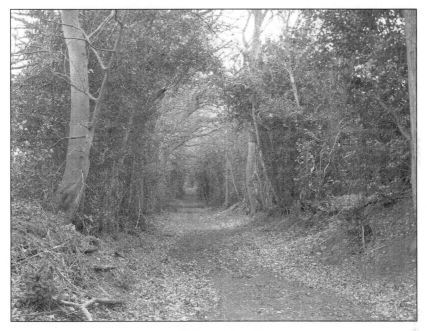

Park Lane, Headley

Pick up instructions for **Walk 7** from point 12 *(see p.40)*.

43

Walk 8 – To Grayshott and back

Distance approximately 6 miles/9.5km (option 3½ miles/5.5km)

This walk starts and ends at the National Trust car park in Pond Road, visiting Ludshott Common, Waggoners Wells, Stoney Bottom, Grayshott and Whitmore Vale. *There is a shorter return route offered from Waggoners Wells visiting Superior Camp – see Walk 8a.*

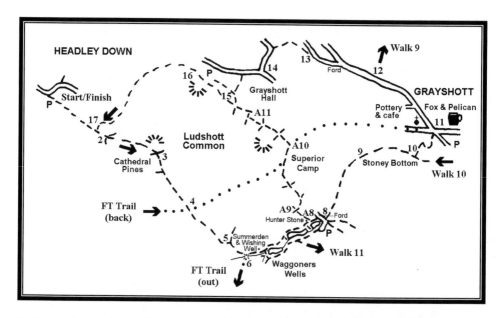

1 From the car park, follow the track up the valley to Ludshott Common.

2 At a junction of several tracks, continue along the centre path which rises between trees for about half a mile past another junction to a crossroads of tracks at the top of the hill with views across the common to the north. This is known locally as 'Charing Cross' (3).

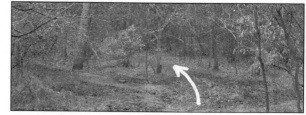

Route at junction of tracks, Point 2

The heathland of the common has been used for Army training during both World Wars – in WW2 activities with tracked vehicles denuded it of most of its vegetation but the trees to the right on this hill, known as 'Cathedral Pines', were protected – however, after the heath fire of May 1980 most of the trees suffered root damage and were later felled.

3 Carry straight on, descending to a valley then rising. Keep straight on where the main track bears left, and cross a bridleway to meet the track which runs

round the edge of the common.

Note: The return leg of the **Flora Thompson Trail** *from Griggs Green to Grayshott crosses our path here.*

4 Take the footpath straight ahead between holly trees. The path crosses a stile then goes alongside a fence across a field to another stile. Descending sharply through woods, it crosses a private woodland track to meet a bridleway at a stile.

5 Turn right down the bridleway, which soon meets the stream flowing from Waggoners Wells.

6 Do not take the bridge over the stream (where the outward leg of the Flora Thompson Trail goes, see photo p.52) but follow the path ahead to pass the National Trust's wishing well and the wall of *Summerden* on the left.

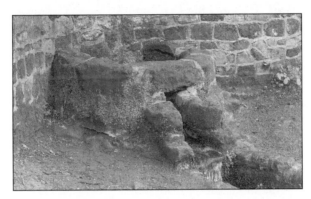

The wishing well below Waggoners Wells

Flora Thompson wrote that at the start of the 20th century, "the local belief was that anyone drinking the water and wishing would have their wish granted, provided they dropped in a pin". *Summerden*, built in 1904, operated as tea-rooms from 1951 for nearly thirty years.

7 Continue uphill to the gate of *Summerden*, then turn right along the side of the valley to arrive at the dam of the bottom pond. From here you may choose paths on either side of the three ponds, crossing at each dam if you wish. *Note:* **Walk 11** *diverges halfway along the south shore of the middle pond.* Eventually you arrive at the ford which crosses the stream running into the top pond. *Note: There is a National Trust car park close by.*

The history of Waggoners Wells (or more correctly Wakener's Wells) is unclear. We believe they were constructed around the 1620s as 'hammer ponds' by Henry Hooke, lord of the manor of Bramshott and a local ironmaster who already had works in Hammer Vale and possibly also in Passfield – but nobody has ever found evidence of industry taking place in this valley. Note the small quarry in the north bank by each dam – it was from here that material was taken to build them, some 400 years ago.

The shorter **Walk 8a** *diverges here – see steps A8–A11 on p.49.*

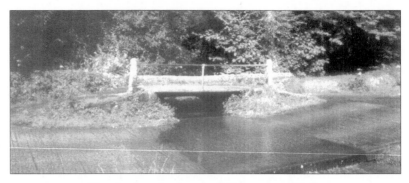

The ford at the head of Waggoners Wells

8 For the full **Walk 8**, follow the footpath up Stoney Bottom – *the start to this is not obvious; cross a ditch a few yards to the right of the photo above.*
Keep left as you enter the mature trees, ignoring the more obvious track ahead, to find the path passing through a small gap in a bank and descending into the valley. This soon passes some more, smaller, ponds.

9 Passing through a barrier by an electricity substation, the path eventually become a track used by local residents' vehicles.

Stoney Bottom is one of the few local valleys whose 'bottom' was not renamed 'vale' in sensitive Victorian times! It was the haunt of heathland workers until the end of the 19th century, particularly the so-called 'broomsquires' who made brooms or besoms from the local chestnut, birch and heather.

10 A few hundred yards after passing a track leading up to the precipitous end of a road on the left, look for a sharp left turn up a concreted road giving vehicular access to the valley for light vehicles. Take this road which winds uphill between houses. At the top, turn left and proceed towards the silver Millennium memorial at the 'Fiveways' crossroads in Grayshott village (11).

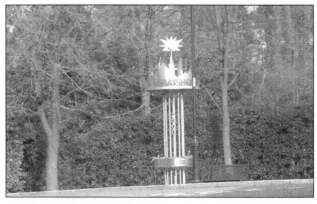

Approaching the Millennium Memorial from Hill Road, Grayshott

Hill Road was named after William 'Body' Hill, a broom-maker who lived in the road and died in 1901 aged 83. This was one of the tracks which

Flora Thompson took to 'escape' into the country when she was assistant post-mistress in Grayshott from 1898–1900. The site of her post office, now demolished, was in Crossways Road where *Pendarvis House* stands (see picture p.77). Grayshott village's two streets offer you many facilities which would be the envy of a small town.

11 You might like to visit the *Fox & Pelican* pub, seen from the crossroads, as a halfway stopping point. There are also Public Conveniences near here.
To continue the walk, go down Whitmore Vale Road leaving St Luke's church to your left. Follow the road out of Grayshott, descending into a tree-shaded valley with a stream.

Sir Arthur Conan Doyle's first wife and son are buried in St Luke's churchyard – they lived in Hindhead at the time. Also you should not miss the Pottery with its gift shop and café, just to the left off Whitmore Vale Road as it descends to the valley.

12 *Note:* **Walk 9** *turns right after the 'Grayshott/ Hampshire' road sign.*
Follow the road along the valley and take a fork to the left which crosses the stream (a ford in wet weather) and shortly afterwards take a 'byway' which forks uphill also to the left with views through the trees to the valley below.

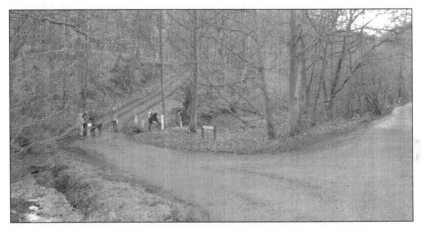

Junction of roads and seasonal ford in Whitmore Vale

13 Follow the bridleway steeply uphill and over a couple of crossing paths – it eventually bears left and joins a road (Hammer Lane). Turn left along the road to its junction with the B3002 opposite the entrance to Grayshott Hall.

Alfred, Lord Tennyson stayed with his family for a year in 1865 at the lowly farmhouse which then stood on the site of Grayshott Hall. Construction of the present Hall began about ten years later and it has been further extended through the years. Owned between 1884–1927 by the Whitaker family, it is now a Health & Fitness Centre.

14 Turn right along the verge of the main road, taking care of fast traffic, and shortly take the bridleway on the left which leaves the road at right-angles

and runs between a boundary fence and the Grayshott Hall grounds to emerge on Ludshott Common. (*Walk 8a rejoins here*).

15 Turn right along the wide sandy track which follows the northern boundary of the Common. Pass the National Trust's 'Dunelm' car park. *Note: there is a map of the common displayed in the car park for those wishing to walk a different route home.* There are good views across to Butser Hill on the South Downs and to the Selborne Hanger.

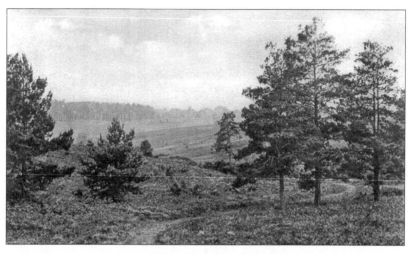

Ludshott Common in 1924

Ludshott Common has belonged to The National Trust since 1908. Along with similar properties in Surrey and West Sussex it forms part of an extensive area of 'lowland heathland' owned by the Trust in this region. Until the early part of the 20th century, the commons were grazed by a variety of different animals which cropped the vegetation and restricted the growth of tree saplings. Since then, this main-tenance has had to be performed by man. The National Trust is carrying out plans to restore endangered species to their natural habitat – these include birds such as the nightjar, woodlark and Dartford warbler and reptiles such as the sand lizard and the smooth snake.

16 Follow the track as it bears gently left leaving the houses of Headley Down on your right, finally zig-zagging in descending to rejoin your outward route.
17 Turn right and follow the track down the valley to your starting point.

ᘒᘒᘒ

Walk 8a – Superior Camp and Grayshott Hall

A8   *Follow **Walk 8** to point 8.*

Take the path from the ford passing to the right of Sir Robert Hunter's stone – this becomes a bridleway rising steeply uphill between old earth banks.

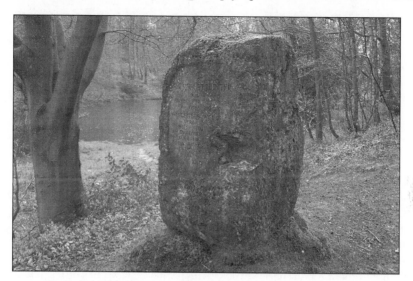

Sir Robert Hunter's memorial stone at Waggoners Wells

Sir Robert Hunter, who lived in Haslemere, founded the National Trust with Octavia Hill and Canon Rawnsley in 1895. He died in 1913, and Waggoners Wells, the first local property to be acquired by the Trust following his death, is dedicated to his memory.

As the track flattens out, note some yards to the left among the trees a banked-up area which is usually covered in stinging nettles – this was the sewage treatment point for Superior Camp (see note below), well illustrating the adage: "nettles grow where man has been".

A9   At a crossways of tracks, turn right. Shortly the track passes through the old perimeter bank (no longer very obvious) of Superior Camp.

Bear left at a fork and then cross a track below an electricity power line. Eventually you pass through a makeshift barrier and onto a concrete road which was at the centre of the old camp. Note some remains of hut foundations still visible to the left of the road here.

Ludshott Common was occupied by the military in 1941, and Superior Camp was constructed by the Canadian Royal Engineers. Note the dates in August 1941 scribed on the top of the concrete cylinders used as road blocks. The Camp was vacated by troops in June 1946, but occupied by squatters. In 1958 all properties were vacated and demolished when empty, and the area was cleared finally in 1964. You may notice some garden plants and hedges which have grown wild here since that time.

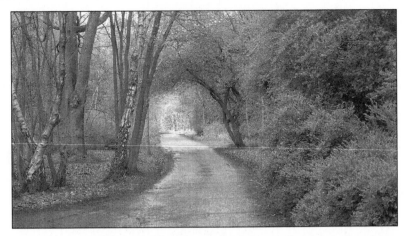

Concrete road through Superior Camp

A10 Just before the road bends to the right, and opposite a privet hedge which has gone wild, take a track to the left. This passes an open area on the right which used to be the camp's parade ground and emerges from the trees onto the heathland of Ludshott Common. From here there are views to the south. Go straight ahead along a bridle path with views to the Oakhanger satellite tracking 'golf balls' ahead – the track drops to a crossways. Go straight ahead up a lesser track which meets a well-used track at a T-junction. Turn right, then shortly bear left to descend to meet the track passing along the northern perimeter of Ludshott Common. Behind trees to the right are the grounds of Grayshott Hall which has been a health centre since the 1960s.

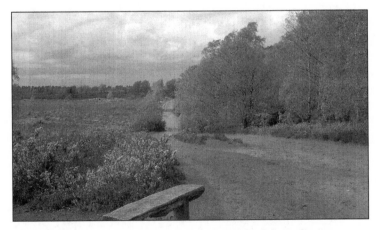

Perimeter track around the north of Ludshott Common

A11 Continue along the perimeter track, which becomes more sandy and wider as it rises to pass the National Trust's 'Dunelm' car park.
(*Here we rejoin **Walk 8** at point 15, see p.48*).

Walk 9 – Three 'new' villages

Distance approximately 8½ miles/13.5km

This walk starts and ends at the National Trust car park in Pond Road and is an extension of Walk 8, visiting the three villages of Grayshott, Beacon Hill and Churt. They are 'new' in so far as before the 1850s there was virtually nothing other than heathland where their centres now stand.

A number of gradients to climb – will take longer than average to complete.

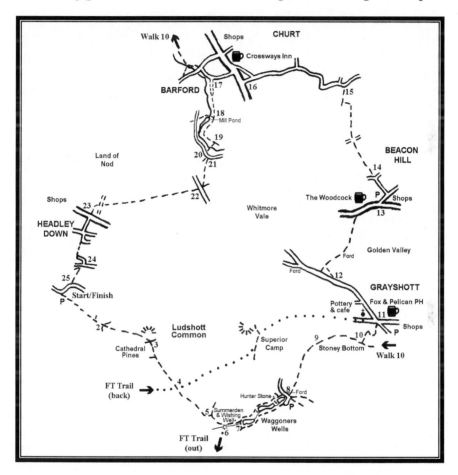

*For notes and illustrations up to point 12, see **Walk 8**.*

1. From the car park, follow the track up the valley to Ludshott Common.
2. At a junction of several tracks (see photo p.44), continue along the centre path which rises between trees for about half a mile past another junction to a crossroads of tracks at the top of the hill with views in winter across the common to the north. This is known locally as 'Charing Cross'.

3   Carry straight on, descending to a valley then rising. Keep straight on where the main track bears left, and cross a bridleway to meet the track which runs round the edge of the common.

4   Take the footpath straight ahead between holly trees. The path crosses a stile then goes alongside a fence across a field to another stile. Descending sharply through woods, it crosses a private woodland track to meet a bridleway at a stile.

5   Turn right down the bridleway, which soon meets the stream flowing from Waggoners Wells.

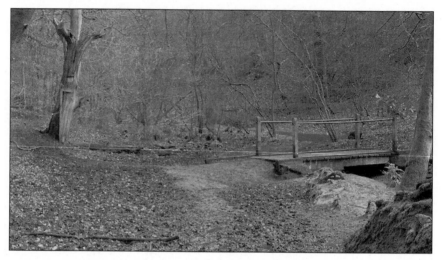

Bridge over the stream below Waggoners Wells

6   Do not take the bridge over the stream but follow the path ahead to pass the National Trust's wishing well and the wall of *Summerden* on the left.

7   Continue uphill to the gate of *Summerden*, then turn right along the side of the valley to arrive at the dam of the bottom pond. From here you may choose paths on either side of the three ponds, crossing at each dam if you wish. Eventually you arrive at the ford which crosses the stream running into the top pond. *Note: There is a National Trust car park close by.*

8   Follow the footpath up Stoney Bottom – *the start to this is not obvious; cross a ditch a few yards to the right of the ford (see photo on p.46)*. Keep left as you enter the mature trees, ignoring the more obvious track ahead, to find the path passing through a small gap in a bank and descending into the valley. This soon passes some more, smaller, ponds.

9   Passing through a barrier by an electricity substation, the path eventually become a track used by local residents' vehicles.

10 A few hundred yards after passing a track leading up to the precipitous end of a road on the left, look for a sharp left turn up a concreted road giving vehicular access to the valley for light vehicles. Take this road which winds uphill between houses. At the top, turn left and proceed towards the silver Millennium memorial at the 'Fiveways' crossroads in Grayshott village.

11 You might like to visit the *Fox & Pelican* pub, seen from the crossroads. There are also Public Conveniences near here.

To continue the walk, go down Whitmore Vale Road leaving St Luke's church to your left. Follow the road out of Grayshott, descending into a tree-shaded valley with a stream.

12 Immediately after crossing the stream (by the Hampshire/Grayshott road sign), take a fairly indistinct path on the right which rises through woodland keeping the road in view to the left – this a joins a track which in turn passes through a metal gate to join a 'byway open to all traffic'. *This byway is deeply rutted by wheeled vehicles and makes very difficult walking. Instead of using it you are recommended to find a path through the trees to its right and follow this over the brow of the hill to rejoin the byway at the ford in the next valley.*

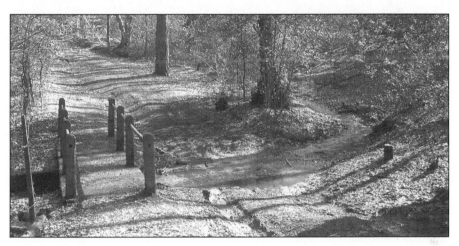

Ford and footbridge where the byway crosses the stream

Follow the byway uphill from the ford for about a third of a mile (there are views to the right across Golden Valley) to meet the A287. Cross the road and turn right along the pavement and past the *Woodcock Inn*, which may offer a welcome rest after all the climbing. Turn left along Beacon Hill Road into the village centre.

The area known as Beacon Hill was, like Grayshott, developed during the second half of the 19th century to service the growing desire of people at that time to come and live in the pure air of the uplands around Hindhead.

13 Pass a parade of shops and turn left down Hill Road. Where the road splits at the bottom take a footpath straight ahead.

14 Follow the footpath downhill (in wet periods it can become a stream) crossing over a forest road and going straight ahead down the valley. This path follows the left side of the valley eventually turning sharp left to meet another footpath – turn right here to descend through a gate to meet a road (Green Lane).

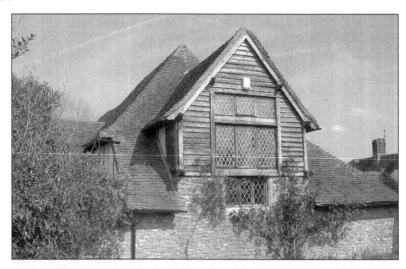

There are several old farmhouses along Green Lane

"All of Churt's old farms are located on the better soils and lie along the Bargate strip from Headley in the west to Thursley in the east. The daunting, hostile areas on either side of the fertile stretch created a natural barrier to development so that Churt remained isolated for centuries." *Olivia Cotton*

15 Turn left and follow Green Lane for about ¾ mile to its junction with the A287. *Note: A right-hand turn here takes you to the centre of Churt village, its shops and pub. Otherwise...*

16 Cross the main road, turn right along the verge then left down Kitts Lane passing old Kitts Farm.

17 At the right-hand bend near the bottom of the hill, turn left to take the track (and public bridleway) serving Barford Mill and the Barracks Cottages.

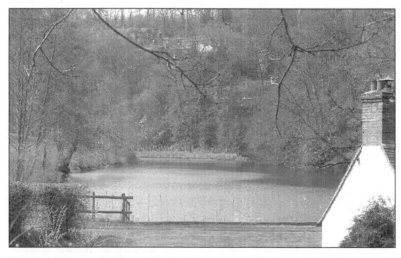

Barford Upper Mill Pond (Power's Pond) from Barracks Cottages

There used to be three watermills on the small stream running down this valley: the upper and lower mills made paper, and the middle one (far older, and generally known as *Barford Mill*) ground corn. The structure of the upper mill no longer exists – the Barracks Cottages were built from its stones.

18 Follow the track past Barford Mill to the upper mill pond.
   Note: You may cross the dam here and take the public footpath on the other side which links to Whitmore Vale Road – follow this along the other side of the valley to meet up at point 20. Otherwise...
19 Carry on up the track and after passing a house on the right (*Easedale*, which used to belong to John Noakes of 'Blue Peter' fame) take the footpath which drops steeply down steps and through a garden gate to cross the stream on a bridge made of railway sleepers. This is the county boundary between Surrey and Hampshire.

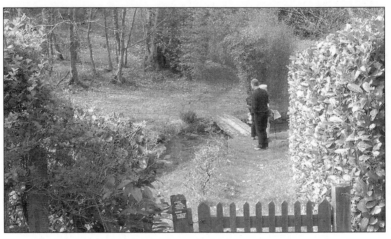

Cross the county boundary through a private garden

Carry on upwards through a landscaped area to meet Whitmore Vale Road.
20 Turn left along the road then, where the road bends left, take the drive to *Walnut Well* on the right.
21 Two footpaths lead off the drive – take the one to the left of the property. This passes along the garden boundary before rising through woods to meet a road (Hammer Lane).
22 Go across Hammer Lane and take the footpath opposite. This leads in a generally straight line through woods, crossing a steep-sided valley and in another half mile or so a tarmac drive (to the *Land of Nod*). After crossing the drive, go straight ahead and shortly turn left through a gap in a fence by a house wall. Cross the end of a cul-de-sac and some open land inside the boundary of the housing estate to reach the main road (B3002).
23 Cross the main road and take Wilsons Road opposite. This leads downhill to Honeysuckle Lane.

Wilsons Road is named after the family who ran the first post office and telephone exchange in Headley Down from their shop, now a private house *The Village Store* at the junction with Fairview Road.

Turn left at the bottom of the hill, and shortly right up Linden Road – at the bend take the footpath straight ahead sharply uphill between a fence and a hedge to arrive at the end of the unsurfaced Oakhill Road. Turn left and follow this as it bears right to meet Furze Vale Road.

24 Go straight ahead here onto a track through the wood.

Note the plaque in the ground to the left of the track as you enter the wood. The 10 acres of 'Openlands' was bought by Dr Elizabeth Wilks (who died in 1953) and is managed for the benefit of local residents by the Headley Public Utility Society.

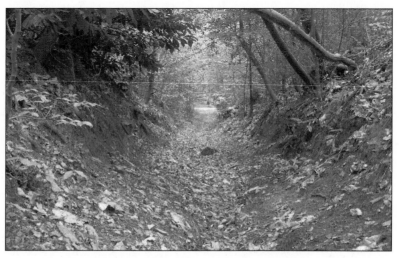

Path down from Openlands to Furze Hill Road

25 Follow the track as it descends, deeply rutted in places, joining Furze Hill Road to arrive back at your starting point.

Walk 10 – Walk with the Devil

Distance approximately 13¾ miles/22km

This walk starts and ends at the National Trust car park in Pond Road, visiting Whitmore Vale, Barford, Frensham Great Pond, the Devil's Jumps, the Devil's Punch Bowl, Hindhead, Tunnel portal, Nutcombe Valley, Miss James' Walk, Stoney Bottom, Waggoners Wells and Ludshott Common.

A number of gradients to climb – will take longer than average to complete.

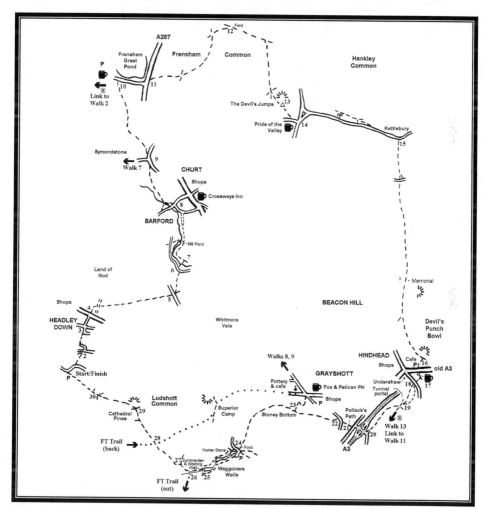

*For notes and illustrations up to point 9, see **Walk 7**.*

1 From the car park, follow Furze Hill Road uphill – where it bends to the right, keep straight ahead on a deep-rutted footpath climbing through woods. Follow this to emerge at a junction of unmade roads.

2 Cross straight over into Oakhill Road – follow this as it bends to the left, and at its dead-end take the footpath to the right and downhill between fence and hedge to join Linden Road as it descends to the bottom of the valley.

3 Turn left along Honeysuckle Lane, and very soon right, up the steep Wilsons Road to meet Grayshott Road.

4 Look for a public footpath sign on the opposite side of the road – take this path, which follows inside the boundary of the housing estate, crossing the end of a cul-de-sac before exiting through a gap in the fence at the bottom left hand corner. Bear right to cross a tarmac drive and take the footpath opposite. This proceeds in a fairly straight line through woods, passing paddocks on the right and some clear land on the left before descending a steep-sided valley, then rising even more steeply up the other side until it meets a road.

5 Cross the road (Hammer Lane) and take the footpath diagonally to the left which descends through woods to Whitmore (or Whitmoor) Vale Road. Turn left for a short distance, then take the footpath to the right.

6 The path descends through a landscaped area to cross the stream on a bridge made of railway sleepers. Climb the steep path on the other side to meet a track running along the side of the valley.

7 Turn left along the track, which soon runs between iron fences and descends passing the sites of three old water mills. Towards the bottom it joins a surfaced road before arriving next to Barford bridge at Churt Road.

8 Cross Churt Road and take the footpath by the water pumping station. This first rises then descends to meet the stream again at a footbridge and ford. Do not cross the stream but turn right to follow the track, which climbs past Ivy Cottage to meet Lampard Lane near Barford Court. Turn left along the lane passing the road to Symondstone (alternatively Simmonstone).
Note: Walk 7 turns left here down the road to Simmonstone.

9 Where Lampard Lane/Star Hill bears right, take a surfaced track straight ahead which becomes a bridle path after the entrance to *Fallowfield Way*. Follow this generally downhill to arrive eventually at the road running along the south side of Frensham Great Pond.

> The pond is not natural, but was created along with several others in the 13th century to provide fish stocks for the Bishops of Winchester. These used to be drained in rotation every five years or so, and barley grown for a season on the exposed bed. It was said that this cleansed it, and prevented growths such as blue-green algae from appearing.

Note: Frensham Pond Hotel lies a few hundred yards to the left along the road which also links to Walk 2 and the 'outer ring'.

10 Turn right along the road to its junction with the main A287 Farnham–Hindhead road.

11 Turn left along the verge, then shortly cross the road to take the bridleway opposite. Walk along this sandy track away from the pond, following number 42 on waymarkers. Pass houses and a pond on the right with King's Ridge on the left before meeting a surfaced road near a footbridge and ford. Turn right and cross the bridge.

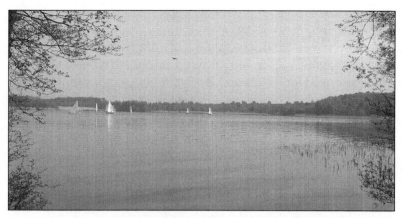

View of Frensham Great Pond from the south shore

12 Go down the road for just over a quarter of a mile, taking the first bridleway (as distinct from footpath) to the right. This passes Axe Pond on the right and heads over flat ground towards and the mounds known as the Devil's Jumps. At a junction, take the footpath which goes straight ahead and eventually up steps to the top of the left-most Jump, from which there is a good view back over Frensham Common.

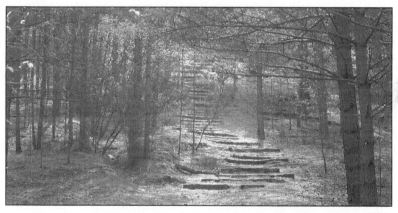

Steps up to the Jumps from the north

There used to be an observatory on top of the middle Jump belonging to Richard Carrington, the eccentric astronomer – this has now gone.

13 From the top of the Jump, take one of the footpaths down the other side, passing between fences to meet a road near the *Pride of the Valley* crossroads.

David Lloyd George lived in this area from 1921 to his death in 1943 – hence the Welsh dragons associated with the Inn. More recently a sculpture park has been opened in the valley opposite.

14 Turn left past the *Pride of the Valley* and cross the main road to take the road opposite signposted Thursley and Elstead. Follow this as it rises slowly. After about a quarter of a mile look for a track on the left (where cars may park) into military land – turn right along a wide, grassy track parallel to the road. At the end of a fence surrounding a house and garden, take a small gate on the right towards the road. Turn left along another track parallel to the road, which it eventually joins by a road-sign to Pitch Place. After a few hundred yards of walking along the road again, take the byway to the right.

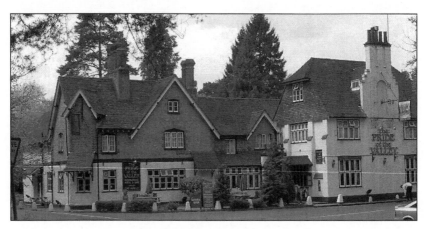

The Pride of the Valley inn

15 Follow the byway as it climbs steadily. Keep right at a fork and then cross straight over a surfaced road. *Note that the track can become very muddy through a sunken section above this point, and there is no alternative path – waterproof footwear recommended.* Through a gate into National Trust land, the track becomes easier as it follows a line of electricity cables uphill. Note the stubby Robertson Memorial to the left just before the track reaches the top of the rise – there are good views from here.

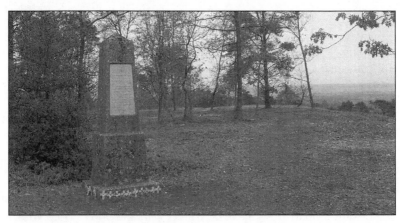

The Robertson Memorial overlooking the Devil's Punch Bowl

Continue along the track as it levels out and crosses a cattle grid. From here, keep to the path following the rim of the Devil's Punch Bowl to arrive at the National Trust car park and café.

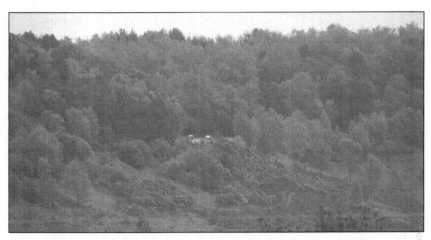

View across the Devil's Punch Bowl to traffic on the A3 in 2005

16 Cross the course of the pre-tunnel A3 road and take the track opposite which skirts the edge of the common to the left of the Devil's Punch Bowl Hotel.

17 After about a hundred yards, look for a gap to the right between garages and go past *Hindhead House* through a small estate to the A287 Hindhead–Haslemere road.

When Hindhead House was built by Professor John Tyndall in 1884 it was the first to be built on Hindhead. He moved here because, according to him, the air on Hindhead was as pure as that

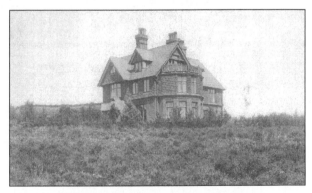

Hindhead House, alone in 1884

in the Alps. Very soon afterwards, and much to his distress, others moved in on hearing this and built houses of their own nearby.

18 Cross the road and pass by a metal barrier into National Trust woodland. Follow the path straight ahead which soon drops steeply into Nutcombe Valley. To your right is the south portal of the A3 Hindhead Tunnel. At a complex of junctions in the valley, turn left then shortly right, up the opposite slope.
*Note: **Walk 13** (the Link to complete the 'outer ring') leaves us to go down the valley at this point.*

19 Follow the path taking forks uphill where possible. This higher part is

known as 'Miss James's Walk', after Miss Marian James who left the land to the National Trust in 1908. The path leaves NT land, passes Fir Cottage and meets a road (Hazel Grove) at a bend. Turn right and follow the path/cycle route past the entrance to the Royal School and across the roundabouts over the A3.

20 Turn left, then shortly right into a National Trust track known as Pollock's Path. Follow this to its end at Crossways Road.

> Sir Frederick Pollock followed John Tyndall's example and moved to Hindhead in 1884, building *Hindhead Copse* (now part of the *Royal School*). He was instrumental in opening and naming the *Fox & Pelican* in Grayshott as a 'Refreshment House' in 1899, but left the district in 1904 considering it had become too crowded. Shortly before his death in 1937, he advised on the form of the Abdication Act.

21 Cross the road, turning right along the pavement then shortly left down Stoney Bottom.

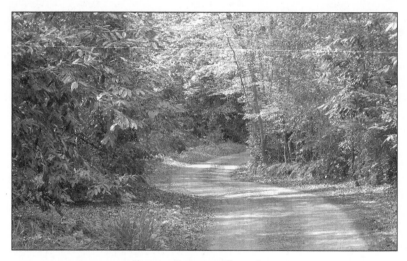

Stoney Bottom, Grayshott

22 Follow the descent of Stoney Bottom valley. After about half a mile, pass a track to the right which leads up to the centre of Grayshott village.

> Note the house called *Broomsquires*. Several of the properties in this area began life as humble dwellings used by makers of brooms, who collected materials from the heath and referred to themselves as 'broomsquires'.

*Note: The route follows **Walk 8** in a reverse direction from this point – see pp.46–44 for notes on this section.*

23 Continue down the valley ignoring tracks to right and left. After passing a barrier by a pumping station the way becomes narrower and sometimes muddy. Eventually the path leaves the bottom of the valley to run along the left-hand bank and passes some small ponds, then it goes over a rise into

woods and down to cross a ditch by the road to the National Trust car park.

24 From here, paths run down both sides of the three Waggoners Wells ponds to the dam of the bottom pond.

25 Keep to the north side at this third dam and follow the path along the valley bank arriving at the house called *Summerden*. The path turns left in front of the garden gate, following the garden wall downwards past the Wishing Well to arrive at a junction by the stream where a track goes left over a footbridge.
*Note: **Walk 14** (the Flora Thompson Trail) leaves us to go across the bridge at this point.*

26 Carry straight on, leaving the stream to the left. The track is usually muddy here. After about two hundred yards take a footpath to the left which goes over a stile into woodland.

27 Follow the footpath across a private woodland track and sharply uphill through trees to a stile at the edge of a field. Cross the field following a fence to another stile, then along a short holly-lined track. The house called *Priors* is to the right.
*Note: **Walk 14** (the Flora Thompson Trail) crosses on its way back to Grayshott at this point.*

28 Our way goes over Ludshott Common. Cross straight over the bridleway here, then over another following a path which dips and eventually rises to a crossing of tracks known as 'Charing Cross'.

29 Carry straight on, ignoring a turn to the right, and descend to a junction of tracks, often muddy.

30 Keep to the valley following the track back to the start point.

Walk 11 – Where Three Counties Meet

Distance approximately 8¼ miles/13km

This walk starts and ends at the National Trust car park in Pond Road, visiting Waggoners Wells, Bramshott Chase, Hammer Vale, Bramshott, Gentles Lane and Gentles Copse.

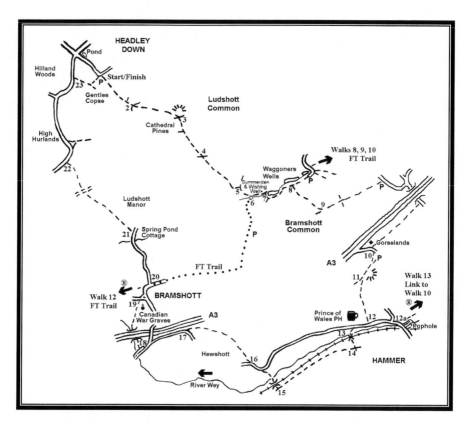

*For notes and illustrations up to point 7, see **Walk 8**.*

1   From the car park, follow the track up the valley to Ludshott Common.
2   At a junction of several tracks (see photo p.44), continue along the centre path which rises between trees for about half a mile past another junction to a crossroads of tracks at the top of the hill with views in winter across the common to the north. This is known locally as 'Charing Cross'.
3   Carry straight on, descending to a valley then rising. Keep straight on where the main track bears left, and cross a bridleway to meet the track which runs round the edge of the common.
4   Take the footpath straight ahead between holly trees. The path crosses a stile then goes alongside a fence across a field to another stile.   Descending

64

sharply through woods, it crosses a private woodland track to meet a bridleway at a stile.

5 Turn right down the bridleway, which soon meets the stream flowing from Waggoners Wells.

6 Do not take the bridge over the stream (where the outward leg of the Flora Thompson Trail goes, see photo p.52) but follow the path ahead to pass the National Trust's wishing well and the wall of *Summerden* on the left.

7 Continue uphill to the gate of *Summerden*, then turn right along the side of the valley to arrive at the dam of the bottom pond. Cross this and turn left along the south bank to pass a second dam. Halfway along the shore of the next pond turn right along a footpath up a wide valley.

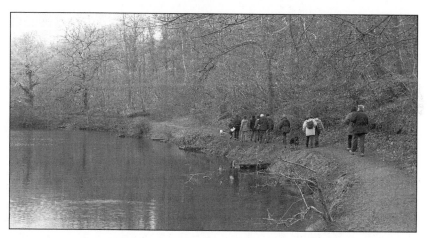

The south bank of Waggoners Wells bottom pond

8 The footpath enters Ministry of Defence lands. Continue up the valley. At a fork after about half a mile bear right and more steeply uphill to meet a track going along the ridge.

9 Turn left along the ridge to enter National Trust land through a gate. Follow the track straight ahead, passing through another gate and a small NT car park. Turn right along the lane here which soon bears left beside the A3 road. Turn right to pass under the A3, then turn right along a track servicing Chase Villas. Follow this past the houses and continue as it enters MoD land and becomes a footpath with garden boundaries to the right until it reaches a lane at Knockhundred Cottage.

> The land on both sides of the Portsmouth Road here was used during the First World War as a camp for Canadian soldiers. The Victorian house next to *Knockhundred Cottage* called *Gorselands*, originally build by Grayshott builder Ernest Chapman for himself, was the HQ. It later became a roadside café. Nearby to the left is the site of the old Seven Thorns Inn.

10 Cross the lane looking for a footpath through bushes opposite – this emerges onto heathland. Follow the wide track below electricity power lines – there

are views to the left across the Wey valley. Look for a footpath signed to the left.

> To the right of the wide track is an area which has been used during two World Wars as a military hospital. The Connaught Hospital, here during the Second World War, was finally closed in 1962.

11 Follow the right of way down into Hammer Vale. It is not very well signed at times – if you fork right at the first parting of the ways and left at the second, you should find yourself on a path which narrows and sinks between gorse bushes before crossing a couple of tracks and passing alongside a hedge to reach a surfaced road.

12 In order to stand with a leg in each of three counties, turn left along the road and follow it for about a quarter of a mile to the point where it crosses the young River Wey.

12a Just after the bridge, take a path to the left into the woodland alongside the river. This rises to a T-junction, joining a path which runs along the top of the old dam which was once part of Pophole Mill. Turn right to cross a footbridge over the channel where a water wheel once worked. It is here that Surrey is to the left of the path, Hampshire to the right, and Sussex straight ahead across the stream. Having experienced this, retrace your steps back to point 12 to continue the walk.

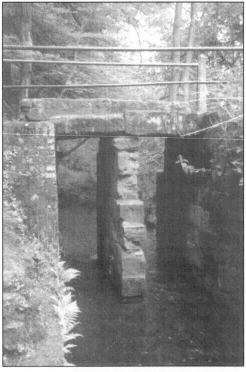

The Northern sluice at Pophole

> Pophole Mill was used until 1776 to make iron. The sluice in the north channel controlled the height of water in the mill pond upstream, which operated a water wheel in the south channel. The wheel was connected to a cam inside the mill building which operated heavy hammers to crush iron ore. It also operated bellows for the hearths where ore was smelted to produce iron ingots.

---

*Note: It is possible to continue from Pophole Mill to Critchmere by turning left at the T-junction and following the path on the Surrey bank of the river, and from there by side roads and tracks up to Hindhead to link with **Walk 10**. See **Walk 13** – 'The Missing Link'.*

---

13 Proceed west along Hammer Lane towards the *Prince of Wales* pub, which is a good mid-point stop. Just before the pub, take a track which forks left off the road and descends beside houses to cross both the river and the railway, the latter on a local level crossing.

14 After crossing the railway and passing through a farmyard, turn right at a gate and stile and follow a bridleway through a field. A hundred yards or so after another gate, fork right along a footpath which follows the railway line, sometimes above and sometimes below it, and joins another bridleway coming in from the left at the top of a hill. Looking right, across the railway line, you can see the ponds of a fish farm. Follow the bridleway past the buildings of *Bridge Farm* to turn right on a track which goes under the railway through a bridge.

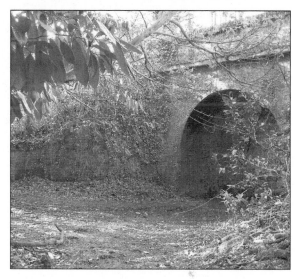

15 Follow the track over the river and uphill to meet a road (Hewshott Lane). Turn left along the road and follow it as it rises and bends left.

16 Turn right along the drive to *Old Barn Farm*. This right of way passes farm buildings and then continues as a narrow path between a hedge on the left and a field fence on the right. Follow this for about half a mile as it crosses stiles and passes a

Bridge taking the track under the railway

house to meet Hewshott Lane again at a bend.

17 Follow Hewshott Lane alongside the A3 trunk road downhill to a junction. Turn left here along a pavement, crossing the road just before a bridge over the river and passing through a gap in the hedge to the old London Road, now a cul-de-sac.

> Just to the north of the road bridge here you can see an old aqueduct which took water in an irrigation channel from one bank of the River Wey to the other.

18 Turn right, and in about a hundred yards left along a footpath (see photo p.84). This path, known locally as 'The Hanger', follows the course of the River Wey under the trunk road and then rises to enter Bramshott churchyard near the Canadian military graves from the First World War (see photo on next page).

> "This path is, and has been from time immemorial, the approach from this side of the parish [of Bramshott] to the Parish Church. A more beautiful or tranquillising approach to a place of worship cannot be imagined..." – Flora Thompson in her *Guide to Liphook*, 1925.

19 Go through the churchyard to the church and exit by the lych gate. Cross over the road and proceed straight ahead to the left of the green triangle. The road bears right passing Limes Close. Shortly, take the next road to the left.

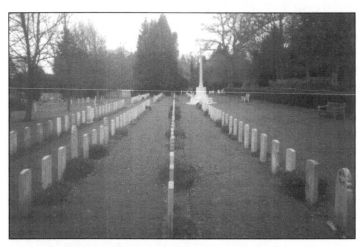

Canadian military graves from WW1 in Bramshott Churchyard

20 The road becomes a sunken lane, dipping down to cross the stream coming from Waggoners Wells before passing *Spring Pond Cottage* on the right.

Note the horse-jump across the stream. This was part of the course which Princess Anne used to ride in the Downlands trials – apparently the language was occasionally colourful at this point!

21 Take the footpath opposite *Spring Pond Cottage*. This rises sharply before crossing fields and a track (with interesting iron steps instead of stiles in a couple of places). Note that the course of the path across the fields is not very obvious – follow the direction of the waymark arrows at the stiles. Ludshott Manor can be seen across fields to the right. The path eventually meets another sunken lane (Gentles Lane).

22 Turn right along the lane and follow uphill as it bears left. After about half a mile at a three-way junction of roads keep right (with Hilland Woods on your left) and after about two hundred yards, just after a house on the right, take a bridleway into Gentles Copse (National Trust) on the right.

23 Follow the bridleway and, where it emerges onto heathland, turn sharp left from the marked way and down a shallow valley to return to the start point.

Walk 12 – To Conford and back

Distance approximately 6 miles/9.5km

This walk starts and ends at the National Trust car park in Pond Road, visiting Ludshott Manor, Bramshott, Conford, Passfield and Waterside.

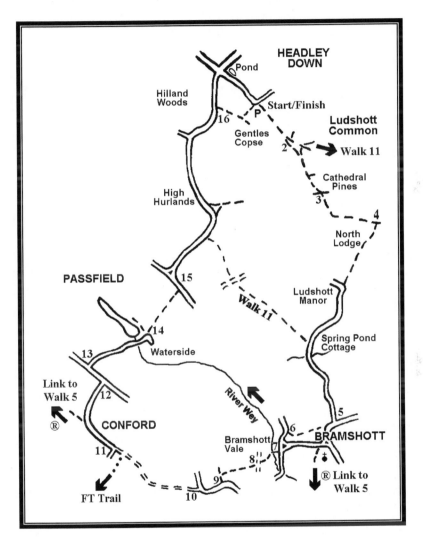

1 From the car park, follow the track up the valley to Ludshott Common.

This valley can become a river at times when flash storms bring water pouring off Ludshott Common. It was particularly bad during and just after WW2 when tank training activity had stripped the common of most of its vegetation. Look carefully and you will see the remains of various concrete constructions designed then to channel the flow.

2 In about a quarter of a mile, look for a track to the right which then bears left to follow the valley before turning right again and uphill beneath overhead electricity cables. Follow this in a fairly straight line along a fire break over the brow of the hill and down to meet another bridleway in a valley.

At the brow of the hill to the left of the track is an area known as 'Cathedral Pines', where the tallest trees on the common once grew.

3 Go almost straight ahead (slightly right) to follow the bridleway (and marked cycleway) which skirts the edge of the common. Turn right at a junction of bridleways to leave the common by a track passing the attractive little North Lodge (4).

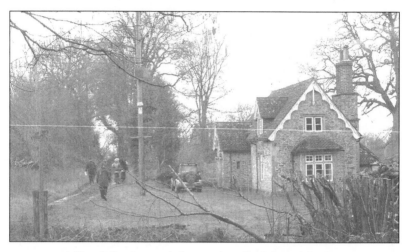

North Lodge and the track to Ludshott Manor

The track you are about to join was once a coach road from Bramshott to London used as an alternative to the what is now the A3. Its course continued across Ludshott Common in a straight line, though now largely overgrown, to emerge at Superior Camp.

4 Follow the track, which becomes a surfaced road at Ludshott Manor, crosses a stream and eventually meets Rectory Lane in Bramshott (5).

Ludshott Manor was rebuilt c.1825 by Sir James Macdonald, Lord of the Manor of Ludshott, and has since been a Carmelite monastery (1954–1968) a Ramana Health Centre (1974–1981) and a retirement home – now converted into private dwellings.

5 *Note: We join* **Walk 14** *(the Flora Thompson Trail from Grayshott to Griggs Green) here until near point 11.*
Turn right and shortly, where the road bears left, continue through some railings and down the sunken path ahead. Here you can imagine how many of the local lanes would have looked in earlier times. At the bottom, turn left onto a road.

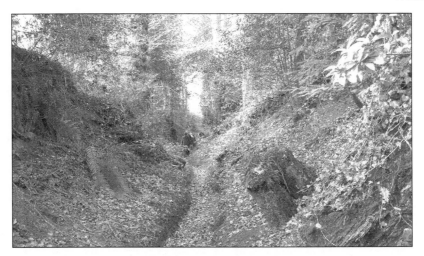

The sunken path at Bramshott

6 Go past the terraces of houses on the right. Note also on your left the house aptly named *Roundabout*, wedged between the forks of the road coming down from Bramshott church – this was once the home of actor Boris Karloff. Continue along the road ahead for a few yards, then right at the gate to *Bramshott Vale*.

There was in the past a shop and post office in the terraced properties. Now Bramshott has none.

7 Walk up the drive and cross over the River Wey. Shortly afterwards, go left through a kissing gate (see photo on next page), cut across a field and go over two stiles towards an avenue of lime trees.

Don't be alarmed at this point to find yourself in the company of some very docile highland cattle. These and other animals are used in season as part of a natural heathland management scheme for local commons, cropping vegetation such as birch, gorse and grass, and allowing the heather to flourish.

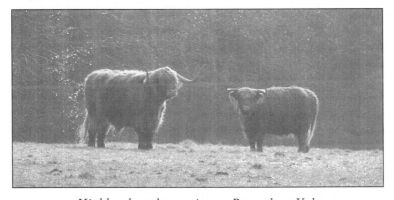

Highland cattle grazing at Bramshott Vale

71

Bramshott Vale House was built in 1732 and was the home of John Butler, ironmaster, who made money from operating furnaces at Pophole (in Hammer) and North Park (in Linchmere).

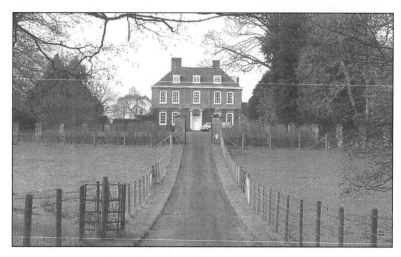

Bramshott Vale house – take the kissing gate to the left

8 Follow footpath signs diagonally across the avenue, through a small metal gate, across a farmyard, over a stile by a larger metal gate and then follow a path along the right-hand side of a field. Turn left at a T-junction of paths and over a stile to meet the B3004 Liphook to Bordon road.

9 Cross carefully and turn right, going along the pavement for about a hundred yards to where the road bears sharp right.

10 Follow the bridleway sign straight ahead down the drive towards *Conford Park House*.
*Note: After slightly more than half a mile **Walk 14** (the Flora Thompson Trail from Grayshott to Griggs Green) leaves us, bearing left at a grass triangle and up the drive of Conford Park House.*

Conford Park House was built by Sir Archibald John Macdonald (who died in 1919), last of the family which held Ludshott Manor for many years. More recently it has been an Ashram.

11 Carry straight on through the hamlet of Conford following the road as it bends right, to meet the B3004 again (12).
*Note: A link to **Walk 5** and the 'Outer Ring' follows the footpath straight ahead in Conford.*

Edge-tools made in Conford by the Moss family were famous for keeping their sharpness. The local school closed in 1964 and is now the Village Hall, owned by the National Trust. The village bakery continued to use the traditional oven method until it stopped trading, much lamented, in 1989.

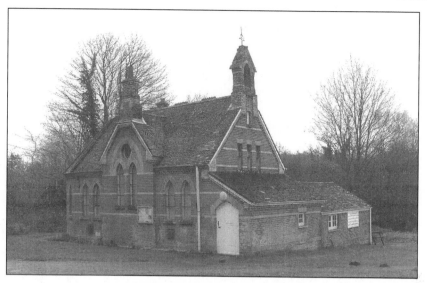

Conford Village Hall (old school)

12 Turn left along the verge, and very shortly take the surfaced drive on the right for *Waterside*.

13 Go down the drive to cross the River Wey at the head of a lake and follow as it curves past the main entrance to a crossroads of tracks. Go straight ahead here along a bridleway.
   Note: **Walk 4** *joins us here for the next mile or so.*

14 Follow the bridleway to Bramshott Lane.

15 Turn left, then shortly right along Gentles Lane which soon becomes a 'sunken lane' climbing uphill. Follow this as it bears left (**Walk 4** *leaves us here*). After about half a mile at a three-way junction of roads keep right (with Hilland Woods on your left) and after about two hundred yards, just after a house on the right, take a bridleway into Gentles Copse (National Trust) on the right.

16 Follow the bridleway and, where it emerges onto heathland, turn sharp left from the marked way and down a shallow valley to return to the start point.

Walk 13 – The Missing Link

Distance approximately 2miles/3.2km

This links Walks 10 and 11 between Hindhead & Hammer, passing through Nutcombe Valley and Critchmere, allowing a complete 'outer ring' walk.

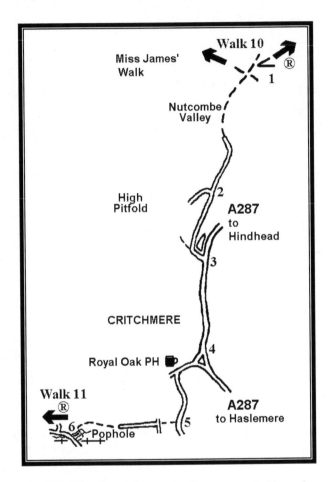

*The link at the Hindhead end begins in Nutcombe Valley where **Walk 10** (at point 19) crosses the valley bottom (see pp.61/62).*

1 Proceed down the valley on the National Trust bridleway track. This passes through a metal gate and becomes a tarred road serving houses on the right. It joins Glen Lea which comes sharply downhill from the right.

2 Continue down the valley on the road (Nutcombe Lane) taking care of motor traffic. In about a quarter of a mile the road turns left, passing the end of a pond, and meets the main A287 Hindhead–Haslemere road.

3 Turn right down the footpath which follows the A287, mercifully at a lower level for most of the way, rising to follow the edge of the road for the last 200 yards before the turning right to Critchmere Hill.

4 Go down Critchmere Hill, then turn left opposite the *Red Lion* public house down Critchmere Lane.

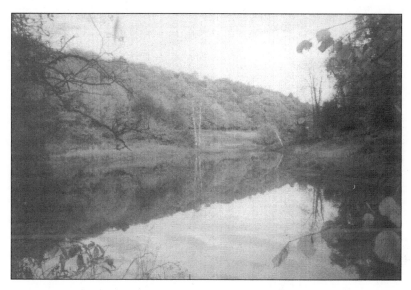

Pond at the bottom of Nutcombe Lane

5 Take the second footpath on the right (opposite Pitfold Close). Cross Pitfold Avenue into Oaktree Lane and follow the footpath at the end of the cul-de-sac leading for about 300 yards beside a cemetery and through woods to the site of Pophole Mill at Hammer. Cross the sluice and turn right to gain the road.

6 Join *Walk 11* at point 12a (see p.66), and continue the 'outer ring' by turning right along the road – this crosses the river and soon bears left towards the *Prince of Wales* public house.

Walk 14 – The Flora Thompson Trail

Distance approximately 10miles/16km

Grayshott to Griggs Green *[Heatherley to Peverel]* and back again

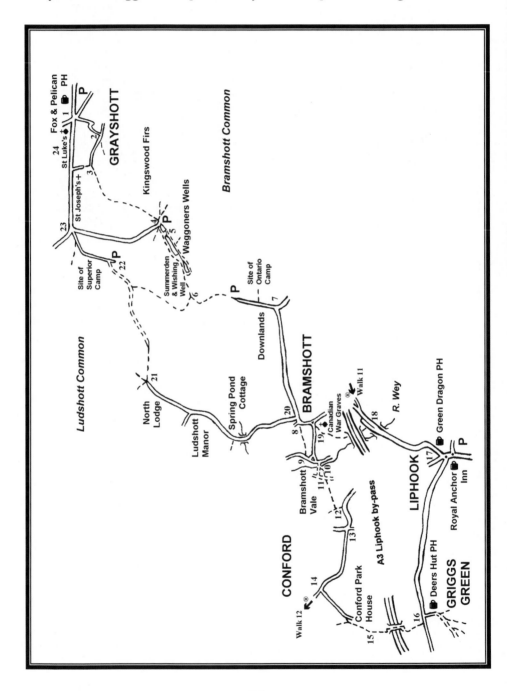

Flora Thompson, author of 'Lark Rise to Candleford', was assistant sub-post-mistress in Grayshott (1898–1900) and later postmaster's wife in Liphook (1916–1928). She loved to take long walks through the countryside, and this trail links the two locations using paths which she would have known well.

෨෨෨

Grayshott to Griggs Green

Distance approximately 5 miles/8km (allow about 2 hours)

Much of the outward route, starting at the *Fox and Pelican* in Grayshott, and ending at the *Deers Hut* in Griggs Green, is little changed from the time Flora herself might have walked it—and both these hostelries are ones which she would have known.

1 From the *Fox and Pelican*, turn right for about 50 yards to the 'Fiveways' crossroads.

To visit the site of Flora's post office, cross over and walk along the right of Crossways Road for about a hundred yards, past the present post office to the property called *Pendarvis House*. The original building here was demolished in 1986.

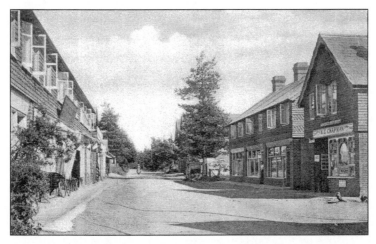

Crossways Road, Grayshott in 1900 – right foreground: Walter G Chapman's post office where Flora Thompson worked at the time

From 'Fiveways,' take the unsurfaced Hill Road, said to be named after broomsquire William 'Body' Hill who lived here in Flora's time. The garden behind the hedge on the right belongs to *Apley House*, built for Edgar Leuchars in 1880. He was the man who pressed for a telegraph service to be installed at Grayshott post office in 1890. At the end, turn right down Stoney Bottom.

This is the nearest of the 'escape routes' which Flora could have used when leaving the post office for a walk in the surrounding countryside. In May 1900, a Dr Coleclough was caught and prosecuted for trying to poison the dog of James Belton, who lived down here – an incident which Flora recalls at some length in *Heatherley*.

2 Turn right at the bottom and proceed down the valley track, which leads towards Waggoners Wells. In a while, note the houses up on the hill to the right. One of these used to be called *Mount Cottage*, and in the late 1870s was a small village shop run by Henry Robinson. It was bought by Mr I'Anson (see below), and Mr Robinson moved to Crossways Road to build a shop there which became the first post office in 1887.

After passing a track which comes steeply down from the right, the land at the top of the hill on the right is the site the first house in Grayshott, built by Edward I'Anson on enclosed common land in 1862 and originally named *Heather Lodge*. [It later became the *Cenacle* convent which was demolished for a housing development in 1999.] Family tradition says that I'Anson rode on horseback from Clapham to view the plot prior to the purchase.

In those days, Grayshott was noted as a lawless area in which gangs of robbers roamed freely, and I'Anson was warned that they would never allow a stranger to settle among them. But he persevered, and he and his family not only lived peaceably, but also began exercise a 'benevolent aristocracy' over the other inhabitants of the growing village, his daughter Catherine becoming particularly active on the parish council and other local organising bodies.

Up on the opposite side of the valley, invisible among the trees, is a house now called *Hunter's Moon*, but originally named *Kingswood Firs*. It was built in 1887 by James Mowatt who was, in a way, instrumental in Flora leaving Grayshott, since it was he who pressed for a rival telegraph service to be established in Hindhead.

3 Keep to the valley path, past a pumping station, and through the wooden barrier. In a while the track moves from the valley floor where this becomes overgrown and boggy, and you pass a series of small ponds before arriving at the top lake of Waggoners Wells.

Before the days of the motor car, the road which crosses the stream here was used as a route for traffic between Haslemere and Frensham.

4 Cross the ford by the footbridge (see photo p.46) and then turn left to follow the path along the right-hand bank of the lake.

Note shortly the stone dedicated to Sir Robert Hunter (see photo p.49), a founder of The National Trust in 1895, who lived in Haslemere and was also employed by the post office, though in a somewhat more senior position than Flora – he was legal advisor at Head Office. Flora would have been aware of a well-reported battle taking place during her time in Grayshott, to protect Hindhead Common. Sir Robert was involved in this, and a few years later initiated a local 'buy-out' to transfer it to the Trust. After his death, Waggoners Wells was also acquired by the Trust, and was dedicated to his memory in 1919. [Note the unusual spelling of 'Waggeners' on it – originally the ponds were called 'Wakeners Wells']

Flora says she 'did not often linger by the lakes' on her Sunday walks, but 'climbed at once by a little sandy track to the heath beyond.' To your right there are several tracks leading uphill to Ludshott Common, and perhaps she met old 'Bob Pikesley' up there or on one of the other local commons, herding his three or four cows.

Also in that direction is Grayshott Hall, site of the old Grayshott Farm rented for several months in 1867 by Alfred Tennyson and his family while building a house of their own near Haslemere. It is said that he wrote his short ode *Flower in the crannied wall* while he was here, some thirty years before Flora trod the same paths.

5 Cross the dam of the top pond, and continue down the left-hand bank of the second pond. Here in autumn, the colour of the trees opposite reflected in the water still brings photographers to the site, as it did in Flora's time.

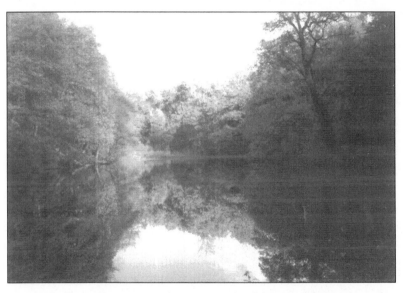

Waggoners Wells – Flora says: 'In autumn the foliage of the trees, red, yellow and russet, was seen in duplicate, above and upon the still, glassy surface.'

The ponds are not natural, having been built in the first half of the 17th century by Henry Hooke, lord of the manor of Bramshott and a local ironmaster. He already had ironworks in the neighbouring Hammer Vale, and presumably wanted to add to his capacity by building another works here. But he seems not to have done so – or at least no evidence of an ironworks has ever been found – and we are left instead to enjoy these quiet pools as his legacy. Flora's husband John used to come fishing here when they lived at Liphook.

The walk may be continued down either side of the third pond, although the path on the left bank is easier. Note the small quarry in the north bank by each dam – it was from here that material was taken to build them, some 400 years ago.

At the dam to the third (and last) pond, take the right-hand side again, and follow the path passing to the left of *Summerden* down to the wishing well.

> When Flora first saw this in 1898 she described it as 'a deep sandy basin fed by a spring of crystal clear water which gushed from the bank above' and said that it had dozens of pins at the bottom which had been dropped in it for luck—some by her. However when she returned in the 1920s, *Summerden* had been built and the water then 'fell in a thin trickle from a lead pipe, the sandy basin having been filled in.' People, she said, seemed to have forgotten its existence.

> She might be happier today to see that it has not quite been forgotten. Although there is no longer a sandy basin, a new well now invites the passer-by to throw in a coin for the benefit of The National Trust – and, of course, to make a wish (see photo p.45).

6 Carry on down the path, cross the stream by the footbridge (see photo p.52), and follow the bridle path to the right and up a sunken track. (In muddy conditions you may wish to take the alternative but steeper route on higher ground). At the crest of the hill keep following this track down and then steeply up the other side of a valley, with the fence of Downlands Estate to your right. In about half a mile, after passing an area used as a car park, the track becomes a paved road.

> To your left is Bramshott Common and the site of Ontario Camp, one of several encampments built in the district by Canadian soldiers during the Second World War. The common had been used extensively by Canadians in the First World War also, and Flora mentions in one of her *Peverel Papers* how 'row upon row of wooden huts, churches, shops and theatres sprang up in a week or two. The whole place became a populous town.' That site is now commemorated by a double row of maple trees along the sides of the A3 Portsmouth road.

> To your right is *Downlands*, which attracted riders such as Princess Anne to the Horse Trials held here annually from 1963 until 1982.

7 After about half a mile, turn right down another paved road (Rectory Lane) and past the main entrance to *Downlands*. The road soon becomes one of the typical 'sunken lanes' of the region before emerging in Bramshott village.

8 Where the paved road bears left, continue through some railings and down the sunken path ahead. Here you can imagine more easily how many of the local lanes would have looked in earlier times (see photo p.71).

9 At the bottom, turn left onto a road. Go past the terraces of houses on the right. Note on your left the house aptly named *Roundabout*, wedged between the forks of the road coming down from Bramshott church. This was once the home of actor Boris Karloff. Continue along the road ahead for a few yards, then right at the gate to *Bramshott Vale*.

10 Walk up the drive and cross the southern River Wey. Shortly afterwards, go left through a kissing gate (see photo p.72), cut across a field and over two stiles towards an avenue of lime trees.

> Don't be alarmed at this point to find yourself in the company of some very docile highland cattle (see photo p.71). These and other animals are used in season as part of a natural heathland management scheme for local commons, cropping vegetation such as birch, gorse and grass, and allowing the heather to flourish. One feels that Flora would have approved.

11 Follow footpath signs diagonally across the avenue, through a small metal gate, across a farmyard, over a stile by a larger metal gate and then follow a path along the right-hand side of a field. Turn left at a T-junction of paths and over a stile to meet the B3004 Liphook to Bordon road.

12 Cross carefully and turn right, going along the pavement for about a hundred yards to where the road bends sharp right.

13 Follow the bridleway sign straight ahead down the drive towards *Conford Park House.*

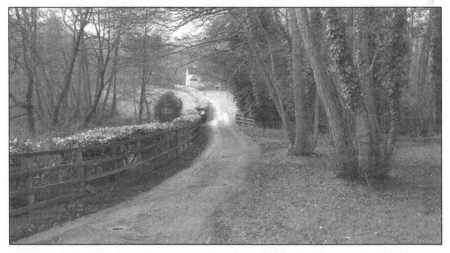

The drive of Conford Park House crossing the bridge towards the gatehouse

14 After slightly more than half a mile, bear left at a grass triangle, cross a bridge by a weir, and pass through some iron gates. Take the footpath to the right, immediately after the gatehouse garden, following behind the line of a hedge. Pass through a smaller iron gate, cross a clearing in front of an old cottage and take the footpath signposted straight ahead. This soon joins a bridleway and winds generally uphill through a beech wood. It can be rather muddy in places.

15 Bear left just before a gate to an Army firing range and follow Bridleway signs across a bridge over the by-pass (which takes the A3 London to Portsmouth traffic away from the centre of Liphook), and eventually down to meet a road (Longmoor Road).

The house called *Woolmer Gate*, to which Flora and her family moved when it was new in 1926, is just along the road to the right.

16 Cross the road and go up the drive almost opposite towards the *Deers Hut* pub and a small cluster of cottages – the original hamlet of Griggs Green.

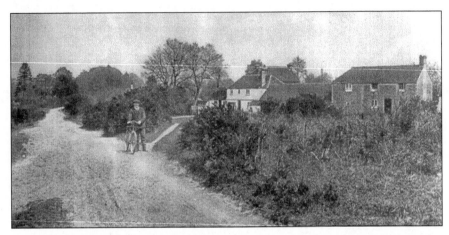

The Deers Hut and cottages as they were at the start of the 20thC

In her 1925 *Guide to Liphook*, Flora says 'it was one of the old forest ale-houses, nor has its function altered much, for neighbours from the scattered houses upon the heath still meet there upon summer evenings to take a glass and discuss things ... just as their forbears must have done for centuries.'

Tracks, once more frequently used, lead from Griggs Green southwards to Forest Mere and beyond, and upwards onto Weaver's Down. This is Flora's *Peverel* – 'a land of warm sands, of pine and heather and low-lying boglands.' She urges you to 'take one of the multitudinous pathways at pleasure; each one leads sooner or later to the summit from which, on a clear day, magnificent views reward the climber. Forest Mere lake lies like a mirror in the woods directly beneath; to the south is the blue ridge of the South Downs; to the north the heathery heights of Hindhead.'

At the end of this section of the guide, Flora adds enigmatically: 'It does not come within the scope of the present work to dwell upon the beauty and interest of this spot more fully; the present writer hopes to deal more fully with it in a future book.' As far as we know, that book never materialised.

See also 'The Peverel Papers' by Flora Thompson, ISBN 978-1-873855-57-7

Return to Grayshott

Distance approximately 5 miles/8km (allow about 2 hours)

There is a lack of convenient public transport between Liphook and Grayshott. For those wishing to make the return journey to Grayshott by foot, here is an alternative which forms a 'figure of eight' with the route out, crossing it at Bramshott.

16 From the *Deers Hut*, turn right along Longmoor Road for the mile-long walk towards the centre of Liphook.

John Thompson and Diana would have cycled to work by this route after they moved to Griggs Green. Along this road also there were one or two small private schools, and Peter Thompson may well have attended one of them. On page 12 of the 1925 *Guide to Liphook*, for example, Miss A. B. Skevington advertises her 'Day School for Girls and Preparatory School for Boys' in a house called *Woodheath*.

17 At the Square take the second road left (London Road) which, before the village was by-passed, bore all the road traffic between Portsmouth and London. On the right-hand side of the road note the HSBC Bank, which was the post office when Flora was here. There is a plaque on the house to its left, where she lived with her family from 1916 to 1926.

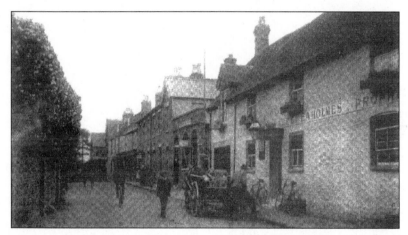

London Road, Liphook around 1914 – the post office is the single-storey building with arched windows; the postmaster's house adjoins it to the left; the 'Green Dragon' is in the right foreground

Further along the road on the right is the old school building now used as a public library. If it is open, you may care to go inside and inspect the sculpture of Flora by Philip Jackson, commissioned in 1981 and moved to the library in 1995.

Follow the left-hand side of London Road out of the village and over the river, following the old road to the left where it divides from the new (18).

Note to the left of the road bridge an old aqueduct over the river, part of a large network of irrigation sluices and channels which stretched for miles along the valley. These were designed to obtain a second annual harvest of animal fodder by flooding the riverside meadows at intervals, and are now part of a conservation project.

18 About a hundred yards after crossing the river, take the footpath to the left. This path, known locally as 'The Hanger', leads into the back of Bramshott churchyard, and was used in Flora's day by Liphook schoolboys attending Bramshott school, the Liphook school being only for girls. In her *Guide to Liphook*, Flora said: 'The raised footpath overhangs, like a terrace, the valley of the infant Wey, a small streamlet at this point, but already known locally as "The River." The path is, and has been from time immemorial, the approach from this side of the parish to the Parish Church.' Its peace has been somewhat shattered in recent years by the construction of the large by-pass bridge overhead.

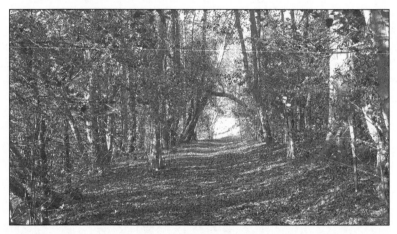

'The Hanger' path between Liphook and Bramshott

On entering the churchyard, you will see to your left the rows of graves of 317 Canadian soldiers who died in the military hospital on Bramshott Common during the First World War – many from the influenza epidemic in late 1918 rather than from enemy action (see photo p.68). Their 95 Catholic colleagues are laid to rest at St Joseph's church in Grayshott, which you will pass later.

On the other side of the churchyard wall, to your right, note the rear of Bramshott Manor which is said to be one of the oldest continually inhabited houses in Hampshire, dating as it does from the year 1220. Flora said: 'Very few houses of its antiquity have escaped so well the hands of the restorer.'

Continue through the churchyard and turn right towards Bramshott church itself ('only five years younger than the Magna Carta') which is well worth a visit.

19 Leave the churchyard by the lych gate, cross over the road and proceed straight ahead to the left of the green triangle. Soon you retrace your steps of the outward journey up Rectory Lane for a few yards. The road bears right passing Limes Close. Shortly, take the next road to the left.

20 Follow this road, which dips down to cross the stream coming from Waggoners Wells, then rises to run past *Spring Pond Cottage* (a favourite of Flora's) and the entrance to *Ludshott Manor* itself.

Where the surfaced road bears left, go straight ahead along an unmade track for another half mile or so. Here, at *North Lodge*, you arrive at the entrance to Ludshott Common, an area of wood and heathland which extends for many hundreds of acres and is now owned by The National Trust.

From this point several routes may be struck at will across the common towards Grayshott. The one detailed below skirts its edge.

21 Go through the wooden posts, and turn right following the bridleway around the edge of the common. It can be boggy in places but this improves when the first of two houses is reached and the track becomes a roughly-surfaced access road. Continue along this, ignoring turns to the right which lead down to the valley of Waggoners Wells.

> In Flora's time, the view to your left would have been open, with purple heather and yellow gorse stretching almost as far as the eye could see. Lack of animal grazing since then has allowed the trees to grow here, but if you walk towards the middle of the common you will find areas which the National Trust has brought back to the original state. And there, as dusk falls on a summer evening, you can still hear the drumming of the Nightjar which so fascinated Tennyson when he lived near here.

22 About half a mile past the houses, you suddenly find yourself on concrete (see photo p.50). This is a remnant of Superior Camp, another of the 'Great Lakes' camps built by the Canadians to house their soldiers during the Second World War. The huts were used as temporary accommodation by local civilians for some years afterwards, but now only a few footings remain, along with the occasional garden plant looking incongruous in a heathland setting.

Turn left and follow the concrete road to its junction with the B3002 Bordon to Hindhead road. *Grayshott House* on your right was once briefly the home of the broadcaster Richard Dimbleby.

23 From here it is a direct walk for about a mile along the pavement and back to Grayshott. In Flora's day this road was described as being 'a sandy track with encroaching gorse'!

> St Joseph's, with the 95 Catholic Canadian graves from the First World War, is on your right about fifty yards along the road next to the driveway to the old *Cenacle* convent, now a gated housing development.

Further along on the right, note the entrance to *Pinewood*, where the I'Anson family lived for many years. The village school and laundry (the latter now a pottery, café and gift shop) which are along School Lane to the left were both

85

institutions started by them.

24 St Luke's church, with its impressive spire, is on your left as you arrive back at the village centre. The foundation stone was laid in the summer of 1898 by Miss Catherine I'Anson, shortly before Flora arrived in the village – the spire was not completed until 1910.

> At the western end of the churchyard are the graves of Conan Doyle's first wife, Mary, and their son Kingsley who died of wounds in the First World War. And at the eastern end, towards the cross-roads, is that of Harold Oliver Chapman and his wife Sarah Annie, born 29 Sep 1878, died 29 Jun 1969. Perhaps you may care to pause here for a while to remember with affection the 'pretty, blue-eyed, sweet-natured girl of eighteen' who, Flora says, made her life tolerable during her time in Grayshott.

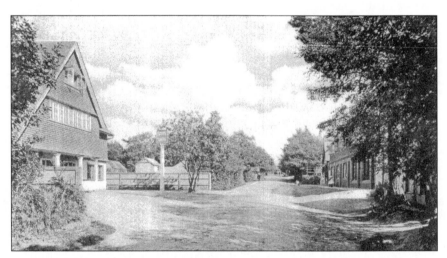

The 'Fox & Pelican' at Grayshott, soon after its opening in 1899

And if you feel weary now after your ten mile walk, then reflect as you relax in the *Fox and Pelican* that Flora would have thought nothing of walking nineteen or twenty miles in one of her daily wanderings!

This walk was first published in 'On the Trail of Flora Thompson'
ISBN 978-1-873855-24-9

The Outer Ring ®

Distance approximately 21½ miles/34.5km

This walk can start at several convenient points, and proceed in a clockwise or anticlockwise direction according to choice.

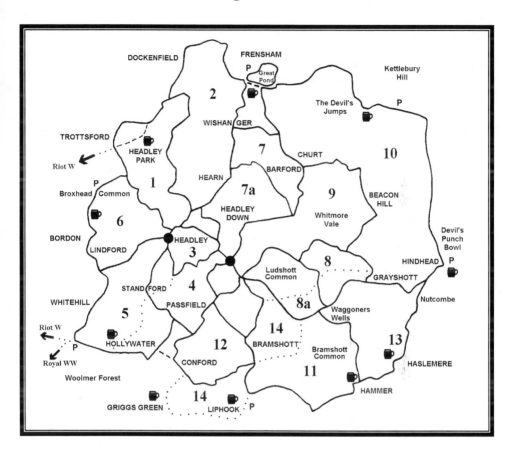

Choice of starting points

There are 'official' car parks on or close to the ring at Frensham Great Pond, Hindhead, and Liphook – but you will find plenty of other places where a car or two may be parked conveniently and some of these are marked on the map above: near Kettlebury Hill, Woolmer Forest and at Broxhead Common. You may also be able to park on request at one of the hotels or pubs on the circuit.

As a suggestion, a starting point at Frensham Great Pond offers convenient mid-point stops at Hammer, Liphook or Griggs Green.

Direction of travel

Instructions for all the walks whose outer parts make up the 'ring' are written in a clockwise direction (except for the lower part of Walk 14, the Flora Thompson Trail, if this is used – see map p.76).

There is, of course, nothing to prevent you from ignoring this convention and doing it withershins!

Mix and Match

You can also construct your own circular walks, for example by linking together Walks 2 & 10, or Walks 11, 12, 5, 6 & 3.

Remember in your planning that walks to the east of our area tend to involve more gradients than those to the west.

Other local walks:—

Footpaths, Bridleways & Byways of Headley Parish

A list and description of all the designated public ways in Headley parish.
Available from Headley Parish Council—01428 713132.

To the Ar and Back

A 'historical stroll' of about a mile around the centre of Headley and Arford.
Details published in a booklet available from The Headley Society or from the publisher of this book.

The Royal Woolmer Way – *shown as 'Royal WW' on maps*

Linear walk of 13 miles/21km from Liss to Frensham.
Details published in a pamphlet available from The Deadwater Valley Trust, The Phoenix Centre, Station Road, Bordon, Hants GU35 0LR.

Walks Around Liphook

Booklet describing 20 circular walks in and around Liphook, and extending into Headley.
Published by the Bramshott & Liphook Preservation Society, 12 London Road, Liphook, Hants GU30 7AN.

Walks through History – at the West of the Weald

A dozen local walks with a historical theme by John Owen Smith, including the Rioters' Walk shown as 'Riot W' on maps in 'Walks Around Headley'.
ISBN 978-1-873855-51-5 December 2006, notes, illustrations and maps.

Walks from the Railway – Guildford to Portsmouth

Circular walks from stations, and linear walks to connect them.
ISBN 978-1-873855-55-3 October 2008, notes, illustrations and maps.

Other books of local interest:—

Headley's Past in Pictures—a tour of the parish in old photographs

Headley as it was in the first half of the 20th century. In this book you are taken on an illustrated tour of the parish by means of three journeys – the first around the centre of Headley and Arford, the second to Headley Down and beyond, and the third along the River Wey and its tributaries.
ISBN 978-1-873855-27-0 December 1999, updated 2003, over 100 photographs, plus historical notes and maps of area.

All Tanked Up—the Canadians in Headley during World War II

A story of the benign 'invasion' of Headley by Canadian tank regiments over a period of four years, told from the point of view of both Villagers and Canadians. Includes many personal reminiscences.
ISBN 978-1-873855-00-3 May 1994, illustrations and maps.

I'Anson's Chalet on Headley Hill—a hidden house, a hidden history

Hidden among the pine trees on Headley Hill there is a Swiss-style chalet. Who built it and why? Judith Kinghorn investigates the history of her house, now called *Windridge*, and discovers a fascinating cast of characters.
ISBN 978-1-873855-48-5 October 2004, illustrated.

The Southern Wey—a guide, by The River Wey Trust

Details of the Southern River Wey from its source near Haslemere through Headley parish to Tilford where it joins the northern branch. Gives fascinating details on the geology, industry, landscape and ecology of our area.
ISBN 978-0-9514187-0-3 reprinted January 1990, well illustrated.

Heatherley—by Flora Thompson—her sequel to the 'Lark Rise' trilogy

This is the book which Flora Thompson wrote about her time in Grayshott.
It is the 'missing' fourth part of her *Lark Rise to Candleford* collection in which 'Laura Goes Further'. Illustrated with chapter-heading line drawings.
ISBN 978-1-873855-29-4 September 1998, notes, illustrations and maps.

On the Trail of Flora Thompson—from Grayshott to Griggs Green

The author has turned detective to discover the true identities behind the pseudonyms which Flora Thompson used for the local places and people she describes in *Heatherley*.
ISBN 978-1-873855-24-9 First published May 1997, updated 2005.

Grayshott—the story of a Hampshire village by J. H. (Jack) Smith

The history of Grayshott from its earliest beginnings as a minor hamlet of Headley to its status as a fully independent parish flourishing on (and across) the borders of Hampshire and Surrey.
ISBN 978-1-873855-38-6 First published 1976, republished 2002, illustr.

Churt: a Medieval Landscape by Philip Brooks

A remarkable insight into the world of ox plough teams, hand-sown crops and a community whose very survival was dependent on the produce of the land.
ISBN 978-1-873855-52-2 First published 2000, republished 2006, illustrated.

John Owen Smith, publisher — www.johnowensmith.co.uk